SLOW COOKER COOKBOOK

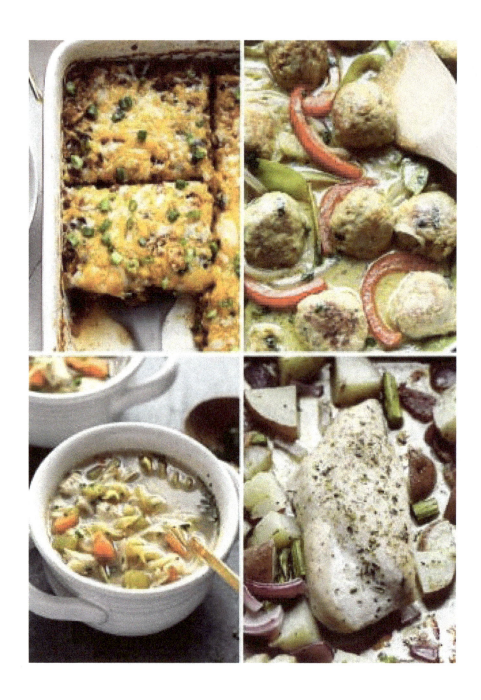

© **Copyright 2021 - All rights reserved.**

The content contained within this book may not be reproduced, duplicated or transmitted without direct written permission from the author or the publisher. Under no circumstances will any blame or legal responsibility be held against the publisher, or author, for any damages, reparation, or monetary loss due to the information contained within this book. Either directly or indirectly.

Legal Notice:

This book is copyright protected. This book is only for personal use. You cannot amend, distribute, sell, use, quote or paraphrase any part, or the content within this book, without the consent of the author or publisher.

Disclaimer Notice:

Please note the information contained within this document is for educational and entertainment purposes only. All effort has been executed to present accurate, up to date, and reliable, complete information. No warranties of any kind are declared or implied. Readers acknowledge that the author is not engaging in the rendering of legal, financial, medical or professional advice. The content within this book has been derived from various sources. Please consult a licensed professional before attempting any techniques outlined in this book. By reading this document, the reader agrees that under no circumstances is the author responsible for any losses, direct or indirect, which are incurred as a result of the use of information contained within this document, including, but not limited to, errors, omissions, or inaccuracies.

SLOW COOKER COOKBOOK FOR BEGINNERS

SLOW COOKER COOKBOOK FOR TWO

SLOW COOKER COOKBOOK FOR BEGINNERS

Table of Contents

Introduction -- **12**

Slow Cooker Meals ------------------------------ **13**

27 Recipes -- **13**

1. Slow-Cooker Chicken Casserole --------------- 13
2. Slow-Cooker Vegetable Lasagna ------------- 15
3. Slow Cooker Bread ---------------------------- 17
4. Slow Cooker Vegetable Stew With Cheddar Dumplings --- 19
5. Slow Cooker Pulled Chicken ------------------ 22
6. Slow Cooker Chicken Chasseur --------------- 24
7. Slow-Cooker Chicken Korma ----------------- 26
8. Slow-Cooker Beef Goulash -------------------- 28
9. Slow Cooker Beef Topside With Red Wine Gravy -- 31
10. Slow Cooked Braised Ribs -------------------- 33
11. Slow Cooker Turkey Pho --------------------- 37
12. Easy Chilli Con Carne ------------------------- 39
13. Slow Cooker Saucy Curry --------------------- 41
14. Slow Cooker Turkey Breast ------------------ 44
15. Slow Cooker Gammon In Cola --------------- 47
16. Slow Cooker Carnitas ------------------------- 50
17. Slow Cooker Chicken Tikka Masala ----------- 52
18. Slow Cooker Pork Loin ------------------------ 54
19. Slow Cooked Beef Stew ----------------------- 56

20. Creamy Black Dhal With Crispy Onions ------ 58

21. Slow-Cooker Ham With Sticky Ginger Glaze - 61

22. Slow Cooker Gingery Chicken ---------------- 63

23. Tender Duck & Pineapple Red Curry --------- 65

24. Slow Cooker Sticky Toffee Pudding ---------- 67

25. Chicken & Red Wine Casserole With Herby Dumplings --- 69

26. Duck With Red Cabbage & Madeira Gravy --- 72

27. Big-Batch Bolognese ------------------------- 76

Conclusion --------------------------------------- **79**

INTRODUCTION

A slow cooker can prove to be useful with a scrumptious feast sitting tight for you and your family by the day's end.

Advantages of Using a Slow Cooker:

Have a supper at home in the slow cooker dispenses with the compulsion to arrange take-out which is frequently not so much nutritious but rather more costly.

Slow cookers normally permit one-venture planning. Putting every one of the ingredients in the slow cooker saves planning time and eliminates cleanup.

Slow cookers are helpful consistently. Rolling in from a virus winter day, the smell of hot soup is inviting. Slow cookers additionally function admirably for mid-year use; they don't heat the kitchen the manner in which an oven may.

Because of the long, low-temperature cooking, slow cookers help soften more affordable cuts of meat.

Slow cooker meals

27 recipes

1. Slow-cooker chicken casserole

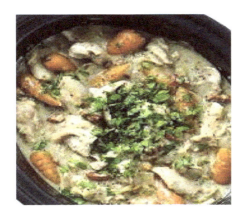

Prep: 10 mins | Cook: 4 hrs. And 15 mins - 7 hrs. and 15 mins| Easy Serves 2 adults + 2 children

Ingredients
- Handle of spread
- ½ tbsp. rapeseed or olive oil
- 1 huge onion, finely chopped
- 1 ½ tbsp. flour
- 650g boneless, skinless chicken thigh filets
- 3 garlic cloves, squashed
- 400g child new potatoes, split
- 2 sticks celery, diced
- 2 carrots, diced
- 250g mushrooms, quartered

- 15g dried porcini mushroom, absorbed 50ml bubbling water
- 500ml stock made with 2 low salt chicken stock 3D shapes (we utilized Kallo)
- 2 tsp. Dijon mustard, in addition to extra to serve
- 2 cove leaves

Strategy
1. Heat a handle of spread and ½ tbsp. rapeseed or olive oil in a huge griddle, cook 1 finely chopped huge onion for 8-10 mins until mollified and beginning to caramelize.
2. In the mean time, put 1 ½ tbsp. flour and somewhat salt and pepper in a bowl and throw 650g boneless, skinless chicken thigh filets in it.
3. Add 3 squashed garlic cloves and the chicken to the pan and cook for 4-5 mins more until the chicken is beginning to brown.
4. Move to your slow cooker, alongside 400g divided child new potatoes, 2 diced celery sticks, 2 diced carrots, 250g quartered mushrooms, 15g dried and splashed porcini mushrooms with the 50ml drenching fluid, 500ml chicken stock, 2 tsp. Dijon mustard and 2 inlet leaves.
5. Give it a decent mix. Cook on Low for 7 hours or High for 4 hours.
6. Eliminate the inlet leaves and present with a little Dijon mustard as an afterthought.

2. Slow-cooker vegetable lasagna

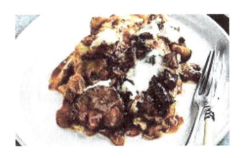

Prep: 30 mins | Cook: 2 hrs. And 30 mins - 3 hrs. | Easy Serves 4

Ingredients
- 1 tbsp. rapeseed oil
- 2 onions, cut
- 2 huge garlic cloves, chopped
- 2 huge courgettes, diced (400g)
- 1 red and 1 yellow pepper, deseeded and generally cut
- 400g can chopped tomatoes
- 2 tbsp. tomato purée
- 2 tsp. vegetable bouillon
- 15g new basil, chopped in addition to a couple of leaves
- 1 enormous aubergine, cut across length or width for greatest surface region
- 6 whole wheat lasagne sheets (105g)
- 125g vegan bison mozzarella, chopped

Technique

1. Heat 1 tbsp. rapeseed oil in a huge non-stick pan and fry 2 cut onions and 2 chopped huge garlic cloves for 5 mins, blending oftentimes until mollified.
2. Tip in 2 diced enormous courgettes, 1 red and 1 yellow pepper, both generally cut, and 400g chopped tomatoes with 2 tbsp. tomato purée, 2 tsp. vegetable bouillon and 15g chopped basil.
3. Mix well, cover and cook for 5 mins. Try not to be enticed to add more fluid as a lot of dampness will come from the vegetables once they begin cooking.
4. Cut 1 enormous aubergine. Lay a large portion of the cuts of aubergine in the base of the slow cooker and top with 3 sheets of lasagne.
5. Add 33% of the ratatouille combination, at that point the leftover aubergine cuts, 3 more lasagne sheets, at that point and the excess ratatouille blend.
6. Cover and cook on High for 2½ - 3 hours until the pasta and vegetables are delicate. Mood killer the machine.
7. Dissipate 125g veggie lover wild ox mozzarella over the vegetables at that point cover and leave for 10 mins to settle and liquefy the cheddar.
8. Dissipate with additional basil and present with a modest bunch of rocket.

3. Slow cooker bread

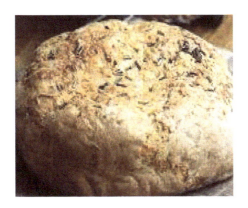

Prep: 15 mins | Cook: 2 hrs. - 2 hrs. and 40 mins | Easy 1 loaf

Ingredients
- 500g solid whole meal flour or solid white flour (or a blend of flours, see tip), in addition to extra for cleaning
- 7g sachet quick activity dried yeast
- 1g fine ocean salt

Strategy
1. Blend the flour, yeast and salt in a huge bowl and make a well in the center. Measure 350ml warm water and empty a large portion of it into the well. Combine the flour and water as one with your fingers or a wooden spoon until consolidated into a somewhat wet, pillowy, useful batter – add a sprinkle more water if important.

2. Tip the batter onto a softly floured surface and massage for at any rate 10 mins until smooth and versatile. This should likewise be possible in a tabletop blender with a mixture snare.
3. Shape the batter into a huge, tight ball and sit the ball on a square of heating material. Utilize the material to lift the mixture into your slow cooker, cover and set the slow cooker to high. Leave for 2 hrs.
4. Lift the bread out using the material. The base ought to be hard and the top ought to be springy, not delicate. (In the event that you have a computerized cooking thermometer, the center of the portion ought to be 90C.) If it isn't prepared, get back to the slow cooker for 15 mins and test again – it could take up to 2 hrs. 30 mins.
5. The bread will not get a critical hull or brilliant tone in the slow cooker. When cooked, you can leave it to cool, or place in the oven at 240C/220C fan/gas 9 for 5-10 mins to get some tone.

4. Slow cooker vegetable stew with cheddar dumplings

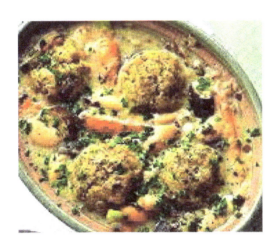

Prep: 20 mins | Cook: 6 hrs. | Easy Serves 6

Ingredients
- 2 tbsp. olive oil
- 200g child carrots , scoured, managed and split assuming huge
- 3 leeks , cut into thick cuts
- 3 garlic cloves , squashed
- 3 tbsp. plain flour
- 400ml vegetable stock
- 2 courgettes , cut into huge lumps
- 2 x 400g jars spread or cannellini beans , depleted and washed
- 1 straight leaf
- 4 thyme , rosemary or tarragon twigs
- 200ml crème fraîche
- 1 tbsp. wholegrain mustard

- 200g wide beans or peas
- 200g spinach
- ½ little pack of parsley, finely chopped, in addition to extra to serve
- For the dumplings
- 100g self-rising flour
- 50g veggie lover suet or cold margarine, ground
- 100g develop cheddar
- ½ little bundle of parsley, finely chopped

Strategy
1. Set the slow cooker to low. Heat 1 tbsp. of the oil in a skillet and fry the carrots for 5 mins until simply brilliant, at that point tip into the slow cooker.
2. Heat the leftover oil in the pan and fry the leeks with a touch of salt for 5 mins until delicate. Add the garlic and mix in the flour. Progressively add the stock, blending, until the flour has broken down and there are no irregularities. Bring to the bubble, at that point tip into the slow cooker. Add the courgettes, beans and spices, beating up with water to cover the veg, if necessary. Cover and cook for 4 hrs.
3. To make the dumplings, tip the flour into a bowl and mix in the suet or margarine until equally conveyed. Add the cheddar, parsley; ½ tsp. broke dark pepper and a touch of salt. Blend in 3-4 tbsp. cold water with your hands to make a delicate, marginally tacky batter (add somewhat more water if necessary). Gap into six and fold into balls.

4. Add the crème fraîche, mustard, expansive beans or peas and spinach to the slow cooker and go it to high. Mastermind the dumplings over the stew, cover and cook for 1-2 hrs. more until firm and multiplied in size. Dissipate with parsley and serve. Will keep for as long as three days in the cooler or in the cooler for as long as a quarter of a year.

5. Slow cooker pulled chicken

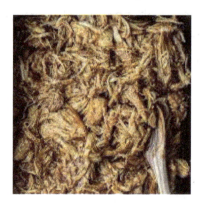

Prep: 5 mins | Cook: 6 hrs. 15 mins| Serves 8-10

Ingredients
- 2 tbsp. vegetable or rapeseed oil
- 10-12 boneless, skinless chicken thighs
- 2 red onions, split and cut
- 2 garlic cloves, squashed
- 2 tsp. paprika
- 2 tbsp. chipotle paste
- 250ml passata
- 100g grill sauce
- 1 tbsp. light brown delicate sugar
- 1 lime, squeezed
- burger buns, taco shells, coat potatoes or rice; coriander leaves; deseeded and cut chilies, and guacamole, to serve (discretionary)

Strategy
1. Heat the slow cooker to low and heat 1 tbsp. oil in a pan. Brown the chicken in clusters, moving it to the slow cooker as you go. Add the excess oil to the pan and fry the onions for 5 mins, or until just relaxed, at that point mix in the garlic and paprika and cook for one more moment. Tip into the slow cooker, at that point whirl 100ml water around the pan and pour this in too.
2. Add the chipotle, passata, grill sauce, sugar and lime juice, at that point season and mix. Cover and cook for 6-8 hrs. until the chicken is truly delicate. Using two forks shred the chicken through the sauce. Serve in buns, taco shells, and coat potatoes or over rice, with coriander leaves, chilies and guacamole, in the event that you like.

6. Slow cooker chicken chasseur

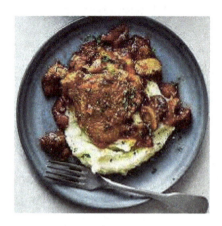

Prep: 15 mins | Cook: 6 hrs. and 35 mins | Serves 2

Ingredients
- 2 tbsp. olive oil
- 4 chicken thighs, skin-on and bone-in
- 2 shallots or 1 onion, finely chopped
- 2 garlic cloves , squashed
- 200g child chestnut mushrooms , split
- 200ml white wine
- 1 tbsp. tomato purée
- 200g chopped tomatoes
- 2 thyme twigs
- 1 inlet leaf
- 400ml hot chicken stock
- little small bunch of parsley , finely chopped, to serve
- squash , coats, pasta or dish potatoes, to serve (discretionary)

Technique
1. Heat the slow cooker to low. Put the oil in a skillet over a medium-high heat. Season the chicken and fry, skin-side down, for 4-5 mins until fresh. Turn and fry for 3-4 mins more until brilliant all finished. Put on a plate and put away.
2. Tip the shallots into the pan and fry for 10 mins over a medium heat until delicate. Add the garlic and mushrooms and fry for 10 mins more until the mushrooms are brilliant. Pour in the wine and air pocket for a couple of moments until decreased significantly. Mix in the tomato purée, chopped tomatoes and spices. Season well and bring to a stew.
3. Tip the sauce into the slow cooker, and top with the chicken thighs (in one layer, if conceivable). Pour over the chicken stock until the chicken thighs are covered, adding somewhat more if necessary. Cover and cook for 6-8 hrs. until the sauce has thickened and the chicken is delicate. Move the chicken to a plate and air pocket the sauce for a couple of moments more with the top off, in the event that you lean toward a thicker sauce (you can possibly do this if there's a diminish work on the slow cooker. If not, empty the sauce into a pan and stew until diminished). Eliminate the skin from the chicken prior to serving, on the off chance that you like.
4. Sprinkle over the parsley and serve the chicken and sauce with rich pound, coats, pasta or little dish potatoes, in the event that you like.

7. Slow-cooker chicken korma

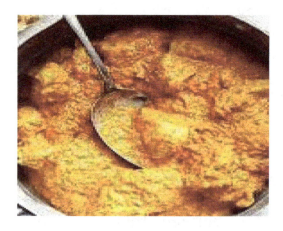

Prep: 15 mins | Cook: 6 hrs. and 20 mins | Serves 4-6

Ingredients
- 2 garlic cloves
- thumb-sized piece ginger, stripped
- 2 huge onions, finely chopped
- 2 tbsp. vegetable oil
- 6 skinless chicken breasts, cut into enormous pieces
- 2 tbsp. tomato purée
- 1 tsp. ground cumin
- 1 tsp. paprika
- 1 tsp. turmeric
- 1 tsp. ground coriander
- ¼-½ tsp. stew powder
- 2 tsp. sugar

- 300ml chicken stock
- 150ml twofold cream
- 6 tbsp. ground almonds
- toasted chipped almonds , coriander, basmati rice and naan breads, to serve (discretionary)

Strategy
1. Heat the slow cooker to low. Put the garlic, ginger and onions in a little blender with a sprinkle of water and whizz to a paste. Heat the oil in a griddle over a medium-high heat and burn the chicken all finished. Eliminate from the pan and put away, at that point add the onion paste. Fry over a medium heat for 10 mins until delicately brilliant.
2. Mix in the tomato purée, flavors, 1 tsp. salt and the sugar, fry for 1 min until fragrant, at that point set the chicken back into the pan (with any resting juices) and add the stock. Mix and bring to a stew, at that point spoon into the slow cooker. Cook on low for 5-6 hrs. until the chicken is delicate and cooked through.
3. Mix through the cream and the ground almonds and air pocket for 10 mins to decrease, if necessary. Disperse with chopped almonds and coriander, in the event that using, present with rice and naans, on the off chance that you like.

8. Slow-cooker beef goulash

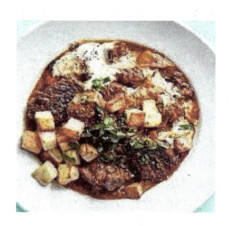

Prep: 25 mins | Cook: 7 hrs. | Serves 8

Ingredients
- 3 tbsp. olive oil
- 2kg braising or stewing steak, cut into lumps
- 2 enormous onions, finely chopped
- 4 blended peppers, cut into 4cm lumps
- 3 garlic cloves, squashed
- 2 tbsp. flour
- 2 tsp. caraway seeds
- 2 tsp. hot smoked paprika
- 1 tbsp. sweet smoked paprika, in addition to extra to serve
- 4 tbsp. tomato purée
- 4 enormous tomatoes cut into little pieces
- 400-500ml meat stock
- 300ml soured cream

- little bundle of parsley, chopped

Technique
1. Heat the slow cooker to low and heat 2 tbsp. oil in a profound griddle over a medium heat. Season and burn the hamburger in clusters until brown on all sides. Move to a plate.
2. Put the leftover oil in the pan and fry the onions for 10 mins until softly brilliant. Add the peppers and garlic, and fry for another 5-10 mins, at that point mix in the flour and the entirety of the flavors. Cook for 2 mins more, at that point mix in the tomato purée, tomatoes and 400ml hamburger stock. Season well. Carry the blend to a stew, at that point tip into the slow cooker with the burned meat. Add the leftover stock, if necessary, to cover the meat totally. Cover and cook for 6-7 hrs. until the meat is delicate and the sauce has thickened marginally.
3. Season to taste; at that point whirl the soured cream and a large portion of the parsley through the stew. Dissipate over the leftover parsley and some sweet smoked paprika, at that point present with little cooked potatoes or brown rice, on the off chance that you like.

9. Slow cooker beef topside with red wine gravy

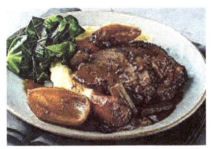

Prep: 20 mins | Cook: 6 hrs. | Plus 1hr marinating | Serves 6

Ingredients
- 1 tbsp. dark peppercorns
- 1 tbsp. English mustard powder
- 2 tbsp. chopped rosemary
- 1 tsp. celery seeds
- 15g dried porcini mushrooms
- 4 tbsp. olive or rapeseed oil
- 1.6kg meat outdoors, cut into 12 cuts
- 600ml hot meat stock
- 1 huge carrot, stripped and generally chopped
- 1 huge onion, generally chopped
- 2 sticks celery, generally chopped
- 2 tbsp. tomato purée
- 200ml red wine
- 1 tbsp. corn flour (discretionary)

Strategy
1. Smash the peppercorns with the mustard, rosemary, celery seeds and a little salt using a pestle and mortar. Barrage the mushrooms to a fine powder in a food processor, at that point mix them in with 2 tbsp. oil and rub everywhere on the meat. Cover and chill for in any event 1 hr., yet overnight is ideal.
2. Heat the slow cooker to high and pour in the stock. Heat 2 tbsp. oil in an enormous pan and brown the meat, at that point put in the slow cooker skin-side up. Fry the carrot, onion and celery in a similar pan over a medium-high heat for around 10 mins. Mix in the tomato purée and wine, scratching the pieces off the lower part of the pan; at that point add this to the slow cooker.
3. Cook on low for 6 hrs; at that point strain the fluid into a pan. Keep the meat and veg covered with foil so they stay warm. Carry the fluid to the bubble; at that point stew until decreased by a third and season. For thicker sauce, blend the corn flour in with 2 tbsp. water and speed into the bubbling fluid. Serve the meat with the sauce, alongside some squash and greens.

10. Slow cooked braised ribs

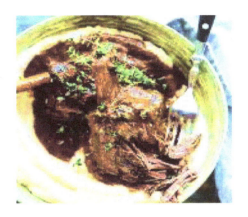

Prep Time: 20 minute | Cook Time: 3 hours 40 minutes | Total Time: 4 hours Yield: 4 servings 1x

Ingredients:
FOR THE SHORT RIBS:
- 4 major, substantial short ribs (around 3 lbs. absolute), overabundance fat managed
- genuine salt and pepper
- 1 tablespoon olive oil
- 1 medium carrot, scoured (no compelling reason to strip), diced
- 1 stem celery, diced
- 1 extremely huge onion, diced
- 6 cloves garlic, finely slashed
- 1 tablespoon tomato glue
- 2 tablespoons flour (utilize a gluten free flour or discard for gf/Paleo)
- 1 ½ cups dry red wine
- 2 cups water

- 2 cove leaves
- 1 enormous twig new thyme (sub ½ teaspoon dried)
- FOR THE CELERY ROOT + PARSNIP PUREE:
- 1 ¼ – 1 ½ lbs. parsnips (3 medium), stripped and cubed
- 1 ¼ – 1 ½ lb. celery root, stripped and cubed
- 4 tablespoons spread (use grass took care of for Paleo)
- ½ – 1 cup entire milk (substitute a nondairy milk for Paleo)
- legitimate salt, to taste
- white pepper, to taste

Directions
1. Remove the short ribs from the cooler, season them liberally on all sides with salt and pepper, and at that point let them sit at room temperature for in any event 30 minutes prior to cooking.
2. Preheat the stove to 325 degrees.* Add olive oil to a huge Dutch broiler over high warmth, at that point painstakingly lay the short ribs down in the hot oil. Let cook until profoundly caramelized (around 5 minutes), at that point turn and earthy colored on every excess side. Try not to surge this progression. Be certain the ribs are bright sautéed on all sides to accomplish the best flavor. Eliminate and let lay on a plate to gather every one of the juices.
3. Channel everything except one teaspoon of oil; at that point add the carrots, celery and onion. Lower the warmth and let cook, mixing

sporadically until mellowed, around 8 minutes. Add the garlic and keep cooking until the vegetables start to scarcely brown, an additional 8 minutes.
4. Add the tomato glue and mix around until it gets caramelized, around 3-4 minutes. Add the flour and cook for 1-2 minutes until it's completely consumed.
5. Add the red wine and go through a wooden spoon to scratch every one of the pieces adhered to the lower part of the container. Add the water, straight leaves and thyme; at that point rise to a bubble.
6. Spot the short ribs back in the skillet alongside their juices, at that point spoon a portion of the fluid and vegetables up and over. Cover and spot in the stove for 1 ½ hours.
7. Skim off any fat that gathers on the top. Flip the short ribs onto the opposite side and add a touch more water to the pot if it's getting dry. Cook for an extra 1 ½ – 2 hours or until the meat is tumbling off the bone. Eliminate from the stove, skim off any extra fat, and at that point let rest in the pot while you make the celery root and parsnip puree.
8. Add the parsnips and celery root to a medium pot and cover with cold water. Rise to a bubble, at that point diminish to a stew and cook until delicate, around 15-20 minutes. Channel and let sit in the colander for a couple of moments to dry (a lot of fluid will make your puree watery).
9. Add the vegetables back to the pot alongside the spread and ½ cup milk. Utilize a drenching

blender to puree until smooth. On the other hand, you can do this in a food processor or blender; however the drenching blender makes it such a ton simpler. I don't suggest hand pounding since you will not get as pleasant of a surface.

10. Add more milk a smidgen at a time to achieve the correct consistency. Season with genuine salt and white pepper to taste. It took an entire tablespoon of salt for mine to taste prepared, so don't be modest (the aggregate sum will rely upon whether you utilized salted margarine and if so which brand).

11. To serve, place a major touch of celery root and parsnip puree on a plate or bowl, top with a short rib and spoon sauce up and over.

12. You can likewise make this formula in a slow cooker. Earthy colored the meat, cook the vegetables, at that point deglaze the skillet with wine and water, at that point move to the slow cooker alongside the meat. Cook on low for 5 hours or until the meat effectively pulls from the bones.

11. Slow cooker turkey pho

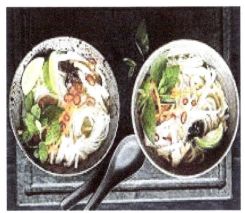

Prep: 20 mins | Cook: 8 hrs. - 10 hrs. | Serves 4

Ingredients
- For the stock
- 50g ginger , thickly cut
- 2 onions , divided
- 3 star anise
- 2 cinnamon sticks
- ½ tbsp. coriander seeds
- 2 cloves
- 1 turkey or chicken corpse, all meat eliminated
- 2-3 tbsp. fish sauce
- 2 tbsp. sugar
- For the pho
- 200g level rice noodles
- 400g cooked and cut turkey or chicken
- 100g beansprouts , whitened, or shredded carrots, mooli or sprouts
- small bunch of Thai basil , mint and coriander leaves
- 2 red chilies , finely cut

- 1 lime, cut into wedges
- hoisin sauce and sriracha sauce, to serve

Strategy

1. Fry the ginger and onion in a dry skillet over a high heat until profoundly shaded. Move to the slow cooker and heat to low. Fry the entire flavors for a couple of mins until fragrant, at that point tip into the slow cooker. Whenever in a rush, basically put in the slow cooker without searing.
2. Add the corpse, at that point pour 3-4 liters bubbling water into the cooker so the bones are covered, guaranteeing you don't pack it. Cover and cook for 8-10 hrs. contingent upon how long you can leave it.
3. Strain the stock, disposing of the bones and flavors. Season with the fish sauce and sugar. To freeze for some other time, leave to cool totally and freeze in a hermetically sealed holder for as long as a quarter of a year. Keep warm in the slow cooker if serving right away.
4. Cook the noodles adhering to pack directions, channel and split between bowls. Top with the turkey and beansprouts or veg, at that point move the stock to a container and pour over enough to fill the dishes (you will have extra, which you can freeze as above). Disperse over the spices and stew, at that point present with the lime wedges and sauces.

12. Easy chili con carne

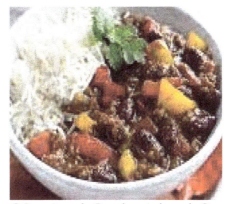

Prep: 20 mins | Cook: 1 hr. | Serves 4

Ingredients
- 2 tbsp. olive oil
- 2 large onions, divided and cut
- 3 large garlic cloves, chopped
- 2 tbsp. gentle stew powder
- 2 tsp. ground cumin
- 2 tsp. dried oregano
- 1kg pack lean minced hamburger
- 400g can chopped tomato
- 2 hamburger stock shapes (we like Just Bouillon)
- 2 large red peppers, deseeded and cut into lumps
- 10 sundried tomatoes
- 3 x 400g jars red kidney beans, depleted

Technique
1. Heat oven to 150C/fan 130C/gas 3. Heat the oil, ideally in a large flameproof goulash, and fry the onions for 8 mins. Add the garlic, flavors and oregano and cook for 1 min, at that point steadily add the mince, blending

admirably until browned. Mix in the tomatoes, add a large portion of a container of water, and at that point disintegrate in the stock and season.
2. Cover and cook in the oven for 30 mins. Mix in the peppers and sundried tomatoes; at that point cook for 30 mins more until the peppers are delicate. Mix in the beans.
3. To serve, reheat on the hob until percolating. Present with avocado or a major serving of mixed greens with avocado in it, some basmati rice or tortilla chips and a bowl of soured cream.
4. On the off chance that you need to utilize a slow cooker, fry your onions in a prospect mins, at that point add your garlic, flavors and oregano and cook briefly. Step by step add the mince until it's brown. Tip into your slow cooker with the tomatoes, peppers, sundried tomatoes and beans; disintegrate in the stock solid shapes and season to taste. Cook on Low for 8-10 hours; at that point fill in as above.

13. Slow cooker saucy curry

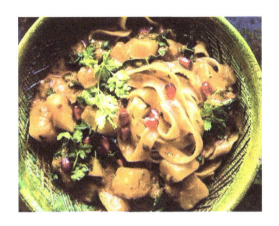

Prep time 15 minutes | Cook time 5 hours | Total time 5 hours 15 minutes | Servings 6 | Calories 382 kcal

INGREDIENTS
- 1/3 cup Thai Red curry paste
- 2 jars (14 ounce) coconut milk
- 1-2 cups low sodium veggie stock
- 1 tablespoon fish sauce
- 1 tablespoon rich peanut butter
- 4 cups cubed butternut squash
- 1 stick cinnamon
- 1 inch new ginger, ground
- juice from 1 lime
- 2 cups destroyed kale
- 1 pound wide egg noodles, like tagliatelle
- 1/4 cup new cilantro, or basil, generally cleaved

- 1 pomegranate, arils for serving

Instructions:
1. In the bowl of your slow cooker, join together the curry paste, coconut milk, 1 cup stock, fish sauce, and peanut butter. Add the butternut squash, cinnamon, ginger, and lime juice. Season gently with salt and pepper. Cover and cook on low for 4-5 hours or on high for 2-3 hours.
2. Mix the kale into the curry and cook 5 minutes until shriveled. Mix in the cilantro (or basil). On the off chance that the curry is excessively thick, add stock to thin.
3. In the mean time, heat a huge pot of salted water to the point of boiling. Heat up the noodles as per bundle directions.
4. To serve, split the noodles between bowls and spoon the curry up and over. Top with pomegranate arils and cilantro. Enjoy!

INSTANT POT
5. In the bowl of your moment pot, consolidate together the curry paste, coconut milk, 1 cup stock, fish sauce, and peanut butter. Add the butternut squash, cinnamon, ginger, and lime juice. Season daintily with salt and pepper. Cover, select the manual setting, and cook on high pressing factor for 8 minutes.
6. When done cooking, utilize the fast delivery capacity and delivery the steam. Set the moment pot to sauté. Mix in the kale and cook 5 minutes until shriveled. Mix in the cilantro (or basil). On the off chance that the curry is excessively thick, add stock to thin.

7. In the interim, heat a huge pot of salted water to the point of boiling. Heat up the noodles as per bundle directions.
8. To serve, split the noodles between bowls and spoon the curry up and over. Top with pomegranate arils and cilantro. Enjoy!

14. Slow cooker Turkey Breast

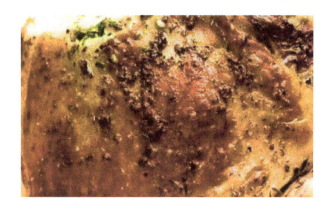

Prep: 15 mins | Cook: 6 hrs. | Total: 6 hrs. 15 mins| serving 8

Ingredients
- - 3 kg/5-6 lb. single turkey bosom , skin on, bone in (Note 1), NOT BRINED
- 1/2 tsp. salt
- Black pepper
- 1 earthy colored onion , split
- 1 head of garlic , divided on a level plane
- 3 branches rosemary, 8 twigs thyme (discretionary)
- Oil , for sprinkling (for skin)
- GARLIC HERB BUTTER (NOTE 2):
- 150 g/10 tbsp. unsalted margarine , mollified
- 1 1/2 tsp. salt

- 1/2 tsp. dark pepper
- 4 enormous garlic cloves, minced
- 1 tbsp. EACH finely slashed new wise, rosemary leaves, thyme leaves and parsley, new
- GARLIC BUTTER GRAVY:
- Chicken stock/stock, for garnish up (whenever required)
- 1/3 cup/50g flour
- 1/2 tsp. + dull soy sauce (or sauce shading) (Note 3)

Guidelines
Garlic Herb Butter: Mix ingredients together.
1. Release skin (video accommodating): Pat bosom dry. Utilize little blade to slice cut on one side to isolate skin from substance. Slide potential gain tablespoon among fragile living creature and skin, all over turkey.
2. Slather: Slather around 2/3 of the margarine under the skin, at that point the leftover everywhere on a superficial level including underside.
3. Season skin: Sprinkle surface with 1/2 tsp. salt + pepper. (Can leave for the time being - 2 days at this stage)
4. Put in Slow Cooker: Place garlic and onion in slow cooker (mine is 5L/5 qt). Spot turkey on top, skin side up. Top with thyme and rosemary twigs.
5. Slow Cook: Cook 6 hours on low, first checking at 5 hours, until inner temperature peruses 165F/75C when embedded into the center.

6. Rest: Transfer turkey to heating plate (save juices). Cover freely with foil, rest for 20 minutes.
7. Fresh: Remove spice twigs, sprinkle turkey with oil (not spread, it consumes/not as firm). Spot under an oven/flame broil on high (~30cm/12" from heat hotspot) for 5 to 10 minutes until skin is firm and tanned - watch out for it, it's speedy.
8. Serve turkey with sauce as an afterthought, or Cranberry Sauce.

Sauce:
9. Strain slow cooker juices into a bowl. Press squeezes out of onion and garlic. In the event that you have under 2.5-3 cups (675-750ml) of fluid, top up with locally acquired stock/stock.
10. At the point when fluid settles, spoon off around 1/4 cup fat/spread from surface.
11. Spot in pan set over medium warmth. At the point when it bubbles, add flour and blend for 1 moment.
12. Add all slow cooker juices into pan. Mix until irregularity free (use whisk if fundamental). Stew for 3 to 5 minutes until it thickens.
13. Add dull soy (if utilizing), pepper and salt to taste. Fill container and present with turkey.
14. Spread Sauce option in contrast to sauce: Pour stressed slow cooker juices into a pan and diminish by about half. Likewise pleasant with a spritz of new lemon juice! Add more spread for extravagance.

15. No water is needed for this, you will be stunned how much fluid is drained by the turkey

15. Slow cooker gammon in cola

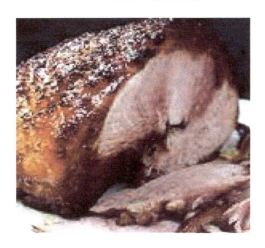

Prep: 10 mins | Cook: 6 hrs. | Serves 6-8

Ingredients
- 1.5-1.8kg unsmoked boneless gammon joint
- 2l cola (not diet)
- 1 carrot, stripped and chopped
- 1 onion, stripped and quartered
- 1 stick celery, chopped
- 1 cinnamon stick
- ½ tbsp. peppercorns
- 1 inlet leaf
- For the coating
- 150ml maple syrup
- 2 tbsp. wholegrain mustard
- 2 tbsp. red wine vinegar

- spot of ground cloves or five-zest

Technique

1. Set your slow cooker to medium. Spot the gammon joint in and cover with the cola. Add 1 chopped carrot, 1 quartered onion, 1 chopped celery stick, 1 cinnamon stick, ½ tbsp. peppercorns and 1 inlet leaf.
2. Cook for 5½ hrs. on low until the gammon is delicate yet at the same time holding its shape, beating up with bubbling water if important to keep the gammon completely covered.
3. Cautiously pour the fluid away, at that point let the ham cool a short time you heat the oven to 190C/170C fan/gas 5. Lift the ham into a simmering tin; at that point remove the skin leaving behind an even layer of fat. Score the fat all over in a confuse design.
4. Blend the maple syrup, mustard, vinegar and ground cloves or five-zest in a container. Pour half absurd, broil for 15 mins, at that point pour over the rest and get back to the oven for another 30 mins.
5. Eliminate from the oven and permit to rest for 10 mins, at that point spoon more coating over the top. Can be simmered on the day or as long as two days ahead and served cold.

16. Slow cooker carnitas

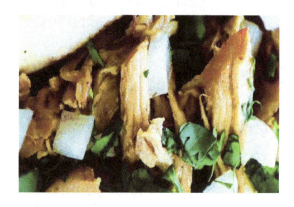

Prep time: 10 Minutes | Cook time: 360 Minutes | Total time: 370 Minutes | Yield: 0 SERVES 6-8

INGREDIENTS
- 1 (4-5 pound) lean boneless pork broil, abundance fat managed, cut into 3-inch lumps
- 1 cup lager (or chicken stock)
- 1 medium white onion, diced
- 4 cloves garlic, stripped and minced
- 1 tablespoon chipotle powder (or 1 chipotle in adobo sauce, minced)
- 2 teaspoons ground cumin
- 1 teaspoon dark pepper
- 1 teaspoon stew powder
- 1/2 teaspoons fine ocean salt

Directions
1. Add all ingredients to a huge slow cooker, and give the blend a mix to join. Cook on low for 6-8 hours or on high for 4-5 hours until the pork

is totally delicate and shreds effectively with a fork.
2. When the pork is cooked, preheat your oven to high warmth and plan two heating sheets with aluminum foil. Utilize a fork to shred the meat into scaled down pieces, and afterward utilize an opened spoon to move it to the readied preparing sheets, spreading the pork in an even layer and giving up the juices in the slow cooker. (Try not to dispose of the juices, we will utilize them later!)
3. Spot one sheet under the grill for around 5 minutes, or until the edges of the pork start caramelizing and crisping up. Eliminate the sheet from the stove, at that point scoop around 1/4 cup of the juices from the slow cooker equally over the pork, and afterward give it a decent throw with some utensils. Sear for an extra 5 minutes to get the meat more firm. At that point eliminate and spoon an extra 1/4 cup of stock over the fresh pork.
4. Rehash with the other heating sheet of pork.
5. Serve quickly in tacos, burritos, plates of mixed greens, or whatever sounds great to you! This pork can likewise be refrigerated in a fixed compartment for as long as 3 days, or frozen in a fixed holder for as long as 3 months.

17. Slow cooker chicken tikka masala

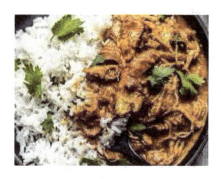

Prep: 20 mins | Cook: 4 hrs. And 30 mins - 7 hrs. and 30 mins | Serves 4

Ingredients
- 8-12 boneless, skinless chicken thighs, each cut into 3 lumps
- 2 tbsp. veg or rapeseed oil
- 1 large onion, chopped
- 2 garlic cloves, squashed
- thumb-sized piece ginger, finely ground or chopped
- 3 tbsp. tikka curry paste
- 500ml passata
- 1 tbsp. tomato purée
- 1 tbsp. malt vinegar
- 1 tbsp. light brown delicate sugar
- 1 cinnamon stick
- 5 cardamom cases
- 100ml twofold cream
- modest bunch chopped coriander

- cooked basmati rice, lime wedges and naan bread, to serve (discretionary)

Technique
1. Heat the slow cooker. Season the chicken, at that point put the oil in a wide griddle and, when hot, add the chicken. Try not to pack the container – you might need to do this in clusters. Cook over a high heat until the chicken is browned, at that point moves it to the slow cooker. Add the onion, garlic and ginger to the skillet and cook for a couple of mins until mellowed. Add a sprinkle of water and scratch any pieces from the lower part of the skillet, at that point tip everything into the slow cooker.
2. Add the leftover ingredients, aside from the cream and coriander, at that point season well and cover with a top. Cook on low for 5-7 hrs. or on high for 4-5 hrs.
3. Add the cream and check the flavoring, adding more vinegar, sugar or salt if necessary. Cook for another 10-15 mins until hot. Scoop among bowls and enhancement with the coriander. Present with rice, naan bread and lime wedges, on the off chance that you like.

18. Slow cooker pork loin

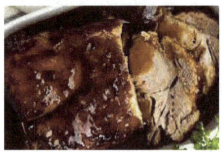

Prep: 30 mins | Cook: 5 hrs. - 6 hrs. | Plus marinade time | Serves 4-6

Ingredients
- 1½ tsp. fennel seeds
- 3 branches new thyme
- 2 garlic cloves
- 2 tbsp. rapeseed or olive oil
- 300g shallots
- about 1.8kg pork midsection, skin eliminated and fat very much scored (cut from the thicker finish of the joint)
- 1 little celeriac, stripped, quartered and cut into pieces
- 2 eating apples, for example, brae burns or coxs, stripped, cored and cut into wedges
- 150ml white wine
- 250ml chicken or pork stock
- 1 tbsp. nectar
- 1 tbsp. Dijon mustard

Technique
1. Delicately squash the fennel seeds with the leaves from the thyme and the garlic in a pestle and mortar. Add 1 tbsp. oil and a lot of salt and pepper; at that point slam to a harsh paste. Rub everywhere on the pork, at that point cover and chill for up to 24 hrs., on the off chance that you have time (2 hrs. if not).
2. Set your slow cooker to a low heat. Pour a kettleful of bubbling water over the shallots, at that point put away for 2 mins until sufficiently cool to deal with – this will make them simpler to strip. Remove the root and eliminate the papery skins. Heat the leftover oil in a large dish or griddle adequately large to fit the pork. Brown the shallots for a couple of mins at that point tip into the slow cooker. Add the celeriac and apples, season well and give them a blend.
3. Brown the pork in a similar dish, on all sides, not failing to remember the closures. Sit on top of the veg and apples, fat-side up, settling the joint in a little so you can fit the top on. Empty the wine into the skillet and air pocket briefly, scratching the lower part of the dish to get any scrumptious pieces. Pour in the stock, nectar and mustard, bubble for another min, and at that point pour over the pork. Cover with a top and cook on low for 5-6 hrs. (contingent upon slow cooker size), turning the pork and blending the veg partially through cooking.
4. Eliminate the pork, enclose by foil and leave to rest for 10 mins prior to cutting to serve close by the veg with cook potatoes and greens.

19. Slow cooked beef stew

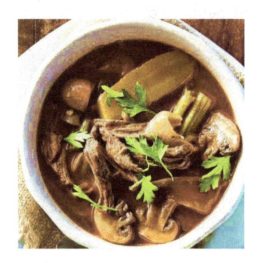

Yields: 8 servings | prep time: 0 hours 20 mins | total time: 8 hours 20 mins

INGREDIENTS
- 2 c. meat stock
- 3 tbsp. generally useful flour
- 2 tsp. Dijon mustard
- 1 lb. carrots, cut into 2-inch pieces
- 1 (8-ounce) bundle cremini mushrooms, divided assuming enormous
- 1 huge red onion, cut into wedges
- 2 huge celery ribs, cut into 2-inch pieces
- 4 cloves garlic, slashed
- 6 branches thyme
- 1 tbsp. canola oil
- 3 lb. pot cook, managed and cut into 4 pieces

- Legitimate salt and newly ground dark pepper
- 1/4 c. tomato glue
- 1 c. dry red wine
- 1 tbsp. unsalted spread
- Hacked new level leaf parsley, for serving
- This fixing shopping module is made and kept up by an outsider, and imported onto this page. You might have the option to discover more data about this and comparable substance on their site.

DIRECTIONS
1. Whisk together stock, flour, and mustard in a 6-quart slow cooker. Add carrots, mushrooms, onion, celery, garlic, and thyme; mix to join.
2. Warmth oil in an enormous skillet over medium-high warmth. Season hamburger with salt and pepper. Cook, turning sometimes, until caramelized on all sides, 10 to 12 minutes. Eliminate to slow cooker. Add tomato glue to skillet and cook, mixing, 1 moment. Add wine and cook, scraping up sautéed bits, 30 seconds; add to slow cooker.
3. Cover and cook until meat is delicate, on low warmth 7 to 8 hours or high for 5 to 6 hours.
4. Dispose of thyme. Eliminate meat and shred with 2 forks; get back to cooker. Mix in margarine.
5. Serve finished off with parsley.

20. Creamy black dhal with crispy onions

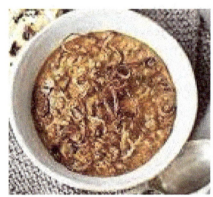

Prep: 35 mins | Cook: 6 hrs. And 35 mins | Plus 4 hrs. Soaking (cook for 2 hrs. 35 mins, if using hob instead of slow cooker)| Serves 4

Ingredients
- 250g dark urid beans (additionally called urid dal, urad dal, dark lentils or dark gram beans - accessible from large stores) - yellow split peas likewise function admirably
- 100g margarine or ghee
- 2 large white onions, divided and meagerly cut
- 3 garlic cloves, squashed
- thumb-sized piece ginger, stripped and finely chopped
- 2 tsp. ground cumin
- 2 tsp. ground coriander
- 1 tsp. ground turmeric
- 1 tsp. paprika
- ¼ tsp. bean stew powder (discretionary)
- little bundle coriander, follows finely chopped, leaves saved to serve

- 400g passata or chopped tomatoes
- 1 fat red stew, penetrated a couple of times with the tip of a sharp blade
- 50ml twofold cream
- To serve
- Cooked rice, naan bread or prepared yams
- Coriander
- Cut red stew
- Lime wedges
- Yogurt (or a twirl of cream)
- Your #1 Indian pickle or chutney
- Fresh serving of mixed greens onions (to make your own, see formula beneath)

Technique

1. Absorb the beans cold water for 4 hrs. (or overnight, on the off chance that you like).
2. Soften the margarine or ghee in a large dish; at that point add the onions, garlic and ginger, and cook slowly for 10-15 mins until the onions are beginning to caramelize. Mix in the flavors, coriander stalks and 100ml water. Fill the slow cooker (or leave in the dish if cooking on the hob). Add the passata and entire red stew. Channel the beans and add these as well, at that point top up with 400ml water. Season well, set the slow cooker to Low and cook for 5-6 hrs. (Or cover and cook for 2 hrs. over an extremely low heat on the hob).
3. When cooked, the dhal ought to be thick and the beans delicate. Mix in the cream, check the flavoring and serve in bowls with naan bread, rice or in a coat potato, with your selection of garnishes. To freeze the dhal, cool totally, at

that point partition into compartments or sandwich packs. Freeze for as long as 2 months, thaw out and heat altogether prior to eating.

FORMULA TIPS
TO MAKE THE CRISPY ONIONS
4. Daintily cut 1 red or white onion. Heat sufficient vegetable or sunflower oil to come 1-2 cm up the side of a large skillet. At the point when hot, fry the onions in bunches until fresh, channel on kitchen paper and sprinkle with salt.

21. Slow-cooker ham with sticky ginger glaze

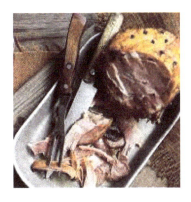

Prep: 20 mins | Cook: 7 hrs. and 20 mins | Serves 6 – 8

Ingredients
- 1 onion, thickly cut
- 10 cloves, in addition to extra for studding
- 1 medium gammon joint, approx. 1.3kg
- 1.5 liter container ginger lager
- 1 tbsp. English mustard
- 3 tbsp. ginger safeguard

Strategy
1. Put the onion and 10 cloves in the base of the slow cooker at that point settle in the gammon joint. Pour over the ginger lager at that point cover and cook on LOW for 7 hours until the gammon is delicate, yet at the same time holding its shape. You can cool at that point cool the gammon at this stage in the event that you like.

2. Heat the oven to 200C/180C fan/gas 6. Cautiously eliminate the skin from the gammon abandoning a layer of fat. Score the fat in a jewel design with a sharp blade, ensuring you don't cut into the meat, at that point stud the focal point of every precious stone with cloves.
3. Blend the mustard and ginger safeguard in a bowl, spoon or brush over the gammon at that point heat for 20 mins until brilliant and tacky. In the event that simmering from cold you should add another 20 mins to the cooking time.

22. Slow cooker gingery chicken

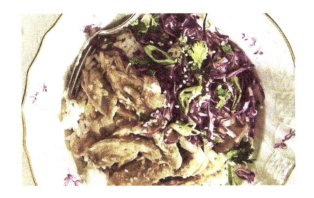

YIELDS: 4 servings | TOTAL TIME: 6 hours 50 mins

INGREDIENTS
- 1/4 c. apricot jam
- 2 tbsp. ketchup
- 1/4 c. soy sauce
- 2 tbsp. grated fresh ginger
- 2 lb. boneless, skinless chicken thighs, trimmed of excess fat
- 4 cloves garlic, chopped
- 1 medium onion, chopped
- 1 small red jalapeño pepper, chopped
- 1/4 c. unseasoned rice vinegar, divided
- Kosher salt and freshly ground black pepper
- 1 c. long-grain white rice
- 1/4 small red cabbage (about 8 ounces), cored and thinly sliced
- 2 scallions, sliced

- 1 tbsp. chopped fresh cilantro, plus more for serving
- 1 tbsp. olive oil
- Toasted sesame seeds, for serving

Instructions:

1. Consolidate apricot jam, ketchup, soy sauce, and ginger in a 5-to 6-quart slow cooker. Add chicken, garlic, onion, and jalapeño; throw to cover. Cook, covered, until chicken is cooked through, 3 1/2 to 4 1/2 hours on high or 5 1/2 to 6 1/2 hours on low. Move chicken to a plate and shred utilizing two forks; get back to slow cooker. Mix in 2 tablespoons rice vinegar. Season with salt and pepper.
2. 25 minutes prior to serving, cook rice as per bundle bearings. Throw together cabbage, scallions, cilantro, oil, and staying 2 tablespoons rice vinegar in a bowl. Season with salt.
3. Serve chicken and sauce over rice finished off with slaw, cilantro, and sesame seeds.

23. Tender duck & pineapple red curry

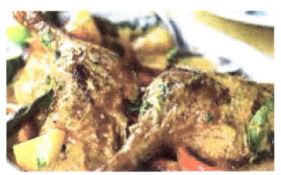

Prep: 20 mins | Cook: 2 hrs. | Serves 6

Ingredients
- 6 duck leg
- 2 tbsp. light brown sugar
- 4 tbsp. red Thai curry paste
- 1 would coconut be able to drain
- 2 tbsp. fish sauce
- 6 kaffir lime leaves
- 1 little pineapple , stripped, cored and cut into pieces
- 1 red stew , deseeded and finely cut, to serve (discretionary)
- Thai basil leaves , to serve (discretionary)

Strategy
1. Heat oven to 180C/160C fan/gas 4. Dry-fry the duck legs in an ovenproof skillet or meal dish on a low heat for a decent 10-15 mins, turning once, until shaded all finished. Eliminate from the dish. Add the sugar to the fat in the

container and cook until caramelized, at that point add the curry paste and cook for not many mins until fragrant. Mix in the coconut milk and a large portion of a jar of water. Stew and mix until everything is joined, at that point add the fish sauce and lime leaves.
2. Slip in the duck legs, cover the dish and cook in the oven for 1½ hrs. until the duck is truly delicate. Lift the duck legs into a serving dish and eliminate fat from the sauce, in the event that you like. The curry can be set up to this stage as long as 2 days ahead and left in the refrigerator, in which case it will be simpler to eliminate the fat.
3. Spot the dish back on the heat, add the pineapple and stew for 2 mins. Change the flavoring, adding more fish sauce for salt, and more sugar for pleasantness. Without a second to spare, mix through a large portion of the stew and a large portion of the Thai basil leaves, assuming using, pour over the duck, disperse with the remainder of the bean stew and basil. Present with jasmine rice.

24. Slow cooker sticky toffee pudding

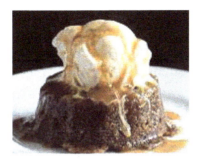

Prep: 30 mins | Cook: 8 hrs. | plus 30 mins soaking | Serves 8

Ingredients
- 250g pitted dates, chopped
- 100g margarine, in addition to extra for the bowl
- 4 tbsp. remedy
- 1 tsp. vanilla concentrate
- 250g light brown delicate sugar
- 300ml twofold cream
- 2 eggs, gently beaten
- 200g self-rising flour
- 1 tsp. bicarbonate of pop
- vanilla frozen yogurt, to serve

Technique
1. Put the dates in a heatproof bowl, cover with 150ml bubbling water, and leave to splash for 30 mins. Spread a 1-liter pudding bowl and line the base with preparing material.

2. Tip a large portion of the margarine, a large portion of the remedy, the vanilla, 75g of the sugar and the cream into a skillet set over a medium heat. Cook for 4-5 mins, blending, until the sugar breaks up. Turn up the heat, bubble for 3 mins, and at that point rush after all other options have been exhausted of salt. Pour 33% of the sauce into the bowl.
3. Beat the excess margarine, remedy, sugar and the eggs together, at that point overlap in the flour, bicarb, ¼ tsp. salt, the dates and their drenching fluid. Spoon into the bowl and smooth the surface, leaving a 1cm hole from the top. Cover with a twofold layer of preparing material and foil, creating a crease in the center so the pod can extend. Secure with kitchen string.
4. Set the slow cooker to low. Sit the bowl inside; at that point add bubbling water so it comes mostly up the bowl. Cover and cook for 7-8 hrs. Run a blade around the edge of the pudding and turn out onto a plate. Reheat the leftover sauce and pore over. Present with frozen yogurt.

25. Chicken & red wine casserole with herby dumplings

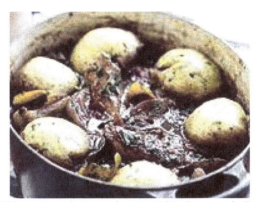

Cook: 50 mins | Ready in 1¾ hours| Serves 6

Ingredients
- 6 section boned chicken breasts or boned for slow cooker (see underneath)
- 3 tbsp. plain flour
- 3 tbsp. olive oil
- 3 onions, each stripped and cut into 8 wedges
- 200g smoked bacon lardons
- 3 garlic cloves, stripped and cut
- 300g large level mushroom, cut
- 2 sound leaves
- 2 tbsp. redcurrant sauce
- 3 pieces of stripped orange zing
- 300ml red wine
- 300ml chicken stock
- For the dumplings
- 100g self-raising flour, in addition to extra for tidying
- 100g new white breadcrumbs

- 1 tbsp. wholegrain mustard
- 140g spread, cubed
- 2 tsp. new thyme leaves, in addition to extra to serve
- 2 tbsp. new parsley, chopped
- 2 egg, softly beaten

Technique
1. Preheat the oven to fan 180C/regular 200C/gas 6. Season the chicken with salt and newly ground dark pepper, at that point coat delicately in a tad bit of the flour. Heat the oil in a large ovenproof lidded goulash dish and, in groups, brown the chicken on the two sides over a high heat. Eliminate the chicken and put away.
2. Lessen the heat, add the onions and lardons and cook for around 5-8 minutes so they are brilliant touched. Add the garlic, at that point sprinkle in the plain flour and cook for 1 moment, mixing to forestall staying.
3. Add the mushrooms, sound leaves, redcurrant sauce and orange zing; at that point pour in the red wine and stock and season with salt and pepper. Bring to the bubble; at that point return the chicken to the goulash dish, ensuring it is all around covered with the fluid. Put on the cover and cook in the oven for 30 minutes.
4. While the goulash is cooking, set up the dumplings. Put one raising flour, breadcrumbs, mustard and margarine in a food processor and rush to a scrap consistency. Add the thyme, parsley, eggs and salt and pepper.

Momentarily rush until the blend frames a genuinely clammy batter. Using floured hands, fold the batter into 6 large, even-sized balls.
5. Eliminate the goulash from the oven when the 30 minutes is up and sit the dumplings on top. Pop the cover back on and get back to the oven for a further 20 minutes, until the goulash is cooked and the dumplings have puffed up. Spoon the chicken and sauce onto six plates and top each with a dumpling. Present with a rich, fruity red wine.
6. On the off chance that you need to utilize a slow cooker, brown the chicken in bunches and move to the slow cooker pot. Add the flour, onions, lardons, garlic, mushrooms, straight leaves, redcurrant, orange zing, red wine and stock, and season. Cover and cook on High for 4 hours. Make the dumplings as per stage 4; at that point sit on top of the dish following 4 hours. Cook for another 1-2 hours, at that point serves.

26. Duck with red cabbage & madeira gravy

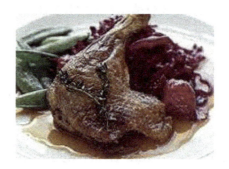

Prep: 3 hrs. And 15 mins - 3 hrs. and 30 mins | Plus overnight salting | Serves 2

Ingredients
- For the duck
- 25g ocean salt drops
- 2 tsp. squashed dark peppercorns
- 4 new cove leaves
- 1 tsp. new thyme leaves in addition to 2-4 branches
- 2 large or 4 little ducks legs (550g/1lb 4oz absolute weight)
- 340g can goose fat
- 300ml/½pint groundnut oil
- For the madeira
- liberal handle of margarine
- 2 shallots , finely chopped
- 1 tsp. plain flour
- 300g tub new chicken stock
- 2 tbsp. madeira
- For the cabbage
- 4 shallots , stripped and divided
- 5 juniper berries , finely chopped

- 400g red cabbage , finely shredded
- 2 tbsp. red wine vinegar
- juice of 1 little orange
- 25g large raisins
- 1 tbsp. redcurrant jam

Technique
1. At any rate 24 hours prior to serving, blend the salt, pepper and spices, aside from the thyme branches, in a large bowl. Add the duck legs and focus on the herby salt until very much covered. Cover and surrender for the time being or to 24 hours in the cooler.
2. Following day, wipe the pungent combination from the duck legs and spot them in a solitary, tight-fitting layer in the base of a skillet. Add the sound leaves from the amaze and pour the goose fat. In the event that it doesn't cover the duck, top up with the groundnut oil. Cook over the least conceivable heat for 2½ hours, so the fat scarcely bubbles. The duck skin ought to be smooth as opposed to brilliant once cooked. Move the legs to a bowl and strain in the fat, pushing the duck under until completely lowered. (The duck would now be able to be chilled and refrigerated for as long as multi month.)
3. While the duck is cooking (or as long as 2 days in front of the supper), make the Madeira sauce and cabbage. For the sauce, dissolve the margarine in a little dish, add the shallots and cook for 6-8 minutes, blending until brilliant. Mix in the flour and cook, blending constantly, until the flour browns – take care not to allow

it to consume. Rush in the stock and keep racing over the heat until somewhat thickened. Add the Madeira and cook for 2 minutes more. Strain through a strainer into a bowl. (The sauce would now be able to be cooled and chilled for as long as 2 days.)

4. For the cabbage, scoop 2 tbsp. of the goose fat from the duck as it cooks (if making at some other point utilize olive oil) and put into a medium skillet. Add the shallots and cook, mixing, until mollified. Tip in the juniper berries and cabbage and cook over a genuinely high heat until the cabbage begins to mellow. Mix in the vinegar, squeezed orange, raisins and redcurrant jam. Cover and leave to cook for 15 minutes, mixing occasionally until delicate. (Cool and chill for as long as 2 days if making ahead.)

5. On the day, preheat the oven to fan 180C/customary 200C/gas 6. Eliminate the duck legs from the fat and wipe away any overabundance with kitchen paper. Put the duck on a wire rack in a broiling tin and top every leg with a twig of thyme. Broil for 10 minutes, at that point add the velvety wild mushroom potatoes to the oven (see formula, underneath) and cook with the duck for 30 minutes, or until the duck skin is brilliant. In the interim, reheat the cabbage and sauce in isolated dish until steaming hot.

6. To serve, put a liberal spoonful of cabbage on serving plates and sit the duck legs on top. Spoon round the sauce and present with the

potatoes. For a green vegetable, rapidly pan sears some sugar snaps.

Formula TIPS

In the event that YOU WANT TO USE A SLOW COOKER...

7. Cook the Madeira and cabbage as above, yet for much more meltingly delicate meat, cook your duck legs in your slow cooker. Salt them for 24 hours as in sync 1 above at that point clear off the salt and spot them in a solitary layer in your slow cooker. Add the thyme, cove and peppercorns and pour over the liquefied fat. Cover and cook on low for 10-12 hours. Move the legs to a bowl and strain the fat at that point complete the process of as indicated by stages 5 and 6 above.

Smooth WILD MUSHROOM POTATOES

8. Hack 8 dried porcini mushrooms (ceps) and put in a large dish with 250ml milk and a 142ml container twofold cream. Add 700g stripped, thickly cut, and washed potatoes. Stew for 8 minutes until the potatoes are practically delicate. Fill a 1 liter ovenproof dish at that point cool and cover. This can be made a day ahead then refrigerated. Put the potatoes in the oven to finish throughout the previous 30 minutes of the duck's cooking.

27. Big-batch Bolognese

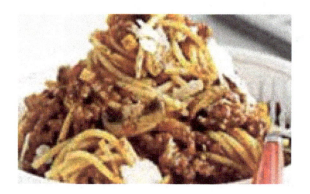

Prep: 25 mins| Cook: 1 hr. and 30 mins | Serves 12
Ingredients
- 4 tbsp. olive oil
- 6 smoked bacon rashers, chopped
- 4 onions, finely chopped
- 3 carrots, finely chopped
- 4 celery sticks, finely chopped
- 8 garlic cloves, squashed
- 2 tbsp. dried blended spices
- 2 narrows leaves
- 500g mushrooms, cut
- 1½ kg lean minced hamburger (or utilize half meat, half pork mince)
- 6 x 400g jars chopped tomatoes
- 6 tbsp. tomato purée
- large glass red wine (discretionary)
- 4 tbsp. red wine vinegar
- 1 tbsp. sugar
- parmesan, to serve

Technique

1. Heat the oil in an exceptionally large pot. Delicately cook the bacon, onions, carrots and celery for 20 mins until brilliant. Add the garlic, spices, cove and mushrooms; at that point cook for 2 mins more.
2. Heat a large griddle until truly hot. Disintegrate in barely enough mince to cover the skillet, cook until brown, at that point tip in with the veg. Keep on browning the mince in groups until spent. Tip the tomatoes and purée in with the mince and veg. Flush the jars out with the red wine, in the event that you have a few, or with a little water, add to the skillet with the vinegar and sugar. Season liberally and bring to a stew. Stew slowly for 1 hr. until thick and sassy and the mince is delicate. Present with pasta and parmesan.
3. In the event that you need to make this in a slow cooker, visit our slow cooker Bolognese formula.
4. Formula TIPS
5. MOROCCAN MINCE
6. Use sheep mince rather than meat, trade the blended spices for 2 tbsp. each ground cinnamon and cumin, and utilize 2 small bunches dried apricots rather than mushrooms.
7. BOLOGNESE BAKE
8. Bubble 2kg potatoes until delicate, channel, at that point squash with 100g margarine and 100g ground cheddar. Spoon the mince between 2 large heating dishes and top with

the squash. Prepare at 200C/180C fan/gas 6 until brilliant and foaming.

Conclusion

I hope you liked all recipes in this book. A slow cooker draws out the flavor in food varieties. A wide assortment of food sources can be cooked in a slow cooker, including one pot dinners, soups, stews and dishes. A slow cooker utilizes less power than an oven. Slow cooked meals are filled with more flavors. You must try these at home and appreciate.

SLOW COOKER COOKBOOK FOR TWO

Table of Contents

Introduction -------------------------------------- **87**

Slow Cooker Meals ------------------------------ **89**

20+ Recipes --------------------------------------- **89**

    1. Braised Pork With Plums --------------------- 89

    2. Cottage Pie ------------------------------------ 92

    3. Golden Veggie Shepherd's Pie --------------- 96

    4. Rich Paprika Seafood Bowl ----------------- 100

    5. Creamy Veggie Korma --------------------- 102

    6. Slow Cooker Lamb Kolifto ------------------ 105

    7. Slow-Cooked Duck Legs In Port With Celeriac Gratin -- 107

    8. Slow-Cooked Greek Easter Lamb With Lemons, Olives & Bay ----------------------------------- 110

    9. Slow-Cooked Celeriac With Pork & Orange 113

    10. Slow Cooker Chickpea Dahl ---------------- 115

    11. Caramelised Squash & Spinach Lasagna --- 118

    12. Lamb Bhuna ------------------------------- 121

    13. Herb-Scented Slow-Roasted Rib Of Beef --- 124

    14. Slow-Roasted Courgettes With Fennel & Orzo-- ---127

    15. Bourbon & Honey-Glazed Brisket With Soured Cream & Chive Mash --------------------------- 130

    16. Sweetcorn Fritters With Slow-Cooked Tomatoes -------------------------------------- 133

    17. Venetian Duck Ragu ------------------------ 136

18. Low 'N' Slow Rib Steak With Cuban Mojo Salsa- --*138*
19. Slow-Roast Pork Rolls With Apple Chilli Chutney -- *141*
20. Beef Bourguignon With Celeriac Mash------ *144*
21. Slow Cooked Ossobuco -------------------- *148*

Conclusion --------------------------------------**151**

INTRODUCTION

A slow cooker can prove to be useful with a tasty feast sitting tight for you and your family toward the day's end.

Slow Cooker Tips and Safety

In the event that you are reluctant to have your slow cooker on and cooking while you are away for the duration of the day, consider cooking food sources during substitute hours that you are home, even while you rest. Cool down the food varieties when they are done cooking, putting away it in the fridge before reheating it in the oven or oven for a feast later.

Here are some fundamental tips and security rules to follow when using a slow cooker:

For simple cleanup and care of your slow cooker, rub within the stoneware with oil or splash it with nonstick cooking shower prior to using it. Slow cooker liners additionally ease cleanup.

Continuously defrost frozen meat and poultry in the fridge prior to cooking it in the slow cooker. To guarantee total cooking, don't place frozen meat in your slow cooker.

Fill the slow cooker no not exactly half full and close to 66% full. Cooking nearly nothing or an excessive amount of food in the slow cooker can influence cooking time, quality and the security.

Since vegetables cook slower than meat and poultry, place the vegetables in the slow cooker first. Spot the meat on top of the vegetables and top with fluid, like stock, water or a sauce.

Add the fluid, like stock, water or grill sauce, recommended in the formula. Since fluids don't reduce away in a slow cooker, much of the time, you can lessen fluids by 33% to one-half while changing over a non-slow cooker formula for slow cooker use.

In the event that conceivable, set your slow cooker on high for the primary hour, and afterward turn the heat setting too low to get done with cooking.

Slow cooker meals
20+ recipes

1. Braised pork with plums

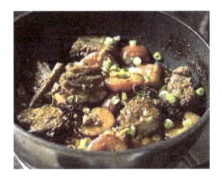

Prep: 25 mins | Cook: 2 hrs. | Plus marinating | Serves 8

Ingredients
- about 1.6kg/3lb 8oz pork shoulder
- 5 tbsp. rice wine
- 5 tbsp. light soy sauce for flavor, 1 tbsp. dull for shading
- liberal thumb-size piece new root ginger
- 5 garlic cloves
- 1 red stew , deseeded and finely chopped
- 2 tbsp. vegetable oil
- pack spring onions , finely cut
- 2 star anise

- 1 ½ tsp. five-flavor powder
- 1 cinnamon stick
- 2 tbsp. sugar , any sort
- 1 tbsp. tomato purée
- 500ml chicken stock
- 6 ready plums , split and stoned

Strategy
1. Cut the pork into huge pieces about the length of your thumb and twice as wide. Put into a bowl or food pack, and add the wine, soy sauces, a large portion of the ginger, a large portion of the garlic and a large portion of the bean stew. Marinate for in any event 1 hr. or up to 24 hrs.
2. Heat oven to 160C/140C fan/gas 3, at that point heat the oil in a large goulash. Tip down the middle the spring onions, staying ginger and garlic, the star anise, five-zest powder and cinnamon. Fry tenderly until fragrant and delicate. Mix in the sugar, turn up the heat, at that point lift the pork from the marinade and turn in the oniony blend for around 3 mins until the meat is simply fixed yet not browned. Tip in the marinade, tomato purée and stock, give it a mix, cover, at that point braise in the oven for 2 hrs.
3. After the main hr. is up, add the plums to the container. Take the cover off and carry on the cooking, revealed. The meat ought to be totally delicate, becoming brilliant brown where it breaks the outside of the sauce. Spoon off any overabundance fat from the surface, at that point scoop the meat and plums

cautiously from the dish with an opened spoon. Turn up the heat and heat up the sauce for 5-10 mins until decreased and somewhat sweet. Return everything to the dish, delicately warm through; at that point disperse the remainder of the spring onions over the top to serve.
4. Formula TIPS
5. In the event that YOU WANT TO USE A SLOW COOKER…
6. Adjust this formula by setting up the pork as indicated by stage 1. At that point cook the spring onions, staying ginger, garlic, stew, cinnamon, star anise, five-zest, and sugar and 2 tbsp. tomato purée. Fry until delicate at that point add the pork, singing until fixed. Put everything into the slow cooker with the marinade and stock, cover and cook for 8-9 hours on Low. Skim off surface fat partially through. Mix in the plums an hour prior as far as possible. Scoop out the plums and meat at that point makes the sauce and serves as per stage 3.

2. Cottage pie

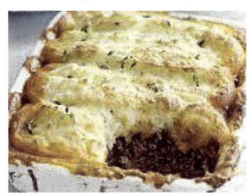

Prep: 35 mins | Cook: 1 hr. and 50 mins | Serves 10

Ingredients
- 3 tbsp. olive oil
- 1 ¼kg hamburger mince
- 2 onions, finely chopped
- 3 carrots, chopped
- 3 celery sticks, chopped
- 2 garlic cloves, finely chopped
- 3 tbsp. plain flour
- 1 tbsp. tomato purée
- large glass red wine (discretionary)
- 850ml hamburger stock
- 4 tbsp. Worcestershire sauce
- not many thyme twigs
- 2 narrows leaves
- For the pound
- 1.8kg potatoes, chopped
- 225ml milk
- 25g margarine
- 200g solid cheddar, ground
- newly ground nutmeg

Technique

1. Heat 1 tbsp. olive oil in a large pan and fry 1¼ kg hamburger mince until browned – you may have to do this in clusters. Put away as it browns.
2. Put the other 2 tbsp. olive oil into the skillet, add 2 finely chopped onions, 3 chopped carrots and 3 chopped celery sticks and cook on a delicate heat until delicate, around 20 mins.
3. Add 2 finely chopped garlic cloves, 3 tbsp. plain flour and 1 tbsp. tomato purée, increment the heat and cook for a couple of mins, at that point return the meat to the container.
4. Pour over a large glass of red wine, if using, and bubble to diminish it marginally prior to adding the 850ml meat stock, 4 tbsp. Worcestershire sauce, a couple of thyme twigs and 2 cove leaves.
5. Bring to a stew and cook, uncovered, for 45 mins. At this point the sauce ought to be thick and covering the meat. Check after around 30 mins – if a ton of fluid remaining parts, increment the heat marginally to lessen the sauce a bit. Season well, at that point disposes of the cove leaves and thyme stalks.
6. In the interim, make the crush. In a large pan, cover the 1.8kg potatoes which you've stripped and chopped, in salted virus water, bring to the bubble and stew until delicate.
7. Channel well, at that point permits to steam-dry for a couple of mins. Squash well with the 225ml milk, 25g margarine, and 3/4 of the 200g solid cheddar, at that point season with

newly ground nutmeg and some salt and pepper.
8. Spoon the meat into 2 ovenproof dishes. Line or spoon on the squash to cover. Sprinkle on the excess cheddar.
9. In the case of consuming straight, heat oven to 220C/200C fan/gas 7 and cook for 25-30 mins or until the garnish is brilliant.
10. On the off chance that you need to utilize a slow cooker, brown your mince in clumps at that point tip into your slow cooker and mix in the vegetables, flour, purée, wine, stock, Worcestershire sauce and spices with some flavoring. Cover and cook on High for 4-5 hours. Make the crush following the past advances, and afterward oven cook similarly to wrap up.

11. Formula TIPS
12. OUR TOP TIPS
13. To get truly smooth, rich squash, utilize a potato ricer or strainer. To stop the pound sinking into the filling, permit the meat to cool prior to garnish with the squashed potato. Freeze in individual ovenproof dishes for a simple supper for one. For a truly fresh, brilliant garnish, streak under the barbecue for a couple of mins prior to serving.
14. Secure FREEZING
15. Ensure the pie is totally cool, at that point cover it well with stick film and freeze. Continuously freeze the pie on the day that you make it. Thaw out in the ice chest short-

term; at that point cook according to the formula. Then again, to cook from frozen, heat oven to 180C/160C fan/gas 4, cover with foil and cook for 1½ hrs. Increment oven to 220C/200C fan/gas 7, uncover and cook for 20 mins more, until brilliant and gurgling.

3. Golden veggie shepherd's pie

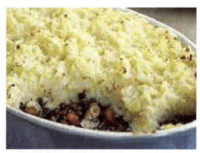

Preparation and cooking time | Prep: 30 mins | Cook: 1 hr. and 45 mins | Serves 10

Ingredients
For the lentil sauce
50g margarine
2 onions, chopped
4 carrots, diced
1 head of celery, chopped
4 garlic cloves, finely chopped
200g pack chestnut mushrooms, cut
2 cove leaves
1 tbsp. dried thyme
500g pack dried green lentils (we utilized Merchant Gourmet Pay lentils)
100ml red wine (discretionary)
1.7L vegetable stock
3 tbsp. tomato purée
For the garnish
2kg floury potato, like King Edwards
85g spread
100ml milk
50g cheddar, ground

Technique

1. To make the sauce, heat 50g spread in a container, at that point tenderly fry 2 chopped onions, 4 diced carrots, 1 chopped head of celery and 4 finely chopped garlic cloves for 15 mins until delicate and brilliant.
2. Turn up the heat, add 200g cut chestnut mushrooms, and at that point cook for 4 mins more.
3. Mix in 2 straight leaves and 1 tbsp. dried thyme; at that point add 500g green lentils. Pour over 100ml red wine and 1.7l vegetable stock – it's significant that you don't prepare with salt at this stage.
4. Stew for 40-50 mins until the lentils are extremely delicate.
5. Season to taste, take off heat, and at that point mix in 3 tbsp. tomato purée.
6. While the lentils are cooking, tip 2kg floury potatoes into a dish of water, at that point bubble for around 15 mins until delicate. Channel well, crush with 85g spread and 100ml milk, at that point season with salt and pepper.
7. To collect the pies, split the lentil combination between every one of the dishes that you are using, at that point top with pound.
8. Dissipate over 50g ground cheddar and freeze for as long as two months or assuming eating that day, heat oven to 190C/fan 170C/gas 5, prepare for 30 mins until the fixing is brilliant.
9. Formula TIPS
10. COOKING INSTRUCTIONS

11. For best outcomes, thaw out the readied pies altogether prior to cooking as expressed. The pies can likewise be cooked from frozen if shy of time – first heat oven to 160C/fan 140C/gas 3, at that point cover the pie with thwart and prepare for 1 hr-1 hr. 20 mins (30 mins for singular pies) until totally delicate when nudged with a blade. Increment the heat to 200C/fan 180C/gas 6, reveal, and at that point keep on cooking for 20 mins until brilliant on top and steaming hot.
12. LENTILS
13. You could likewise utilize three jars of washed and depleted green lentils for this – basically make the stock, at that point stew them for only 10 minutes.
14. Instructions to FREEZE
15. On the off chance that you have bunches of pie dishes, you can make the pies in an assortment of sizes to suit various events, at that point freeze them. I like to make two large pies to serve up to four, in addition to two individual pies – ideal for an independent dinner or a heavenly dinner for the sitter. In the event that you don't have heaps of dishes, you can freeze the sauce, squash and cheddar in isolated cooler sacks, at that point thaw out and gather when required.
16. In the event that YOU WANT TO USE A SLOW COOKER...
17. Fry off your onions, celery, carrots and garlic for 15 mins in a skillet. Tip into your slow cooker with the mushrooms, spices and lentils. Pour over the stock and wine, cover and cook

on High for 5-6 hours. In the mean time make the squashed potato as per stage 6. Mood killer the slow cooker, season and mix in the tomato purée. Proceed from stage 7, splitting the lentils between dishes, top with the pound and cheddar and cook for 30 mins until quite hot.

4. Rich paprika seafood bowl

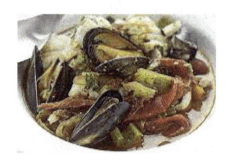

Prep: 10 mins | Cook: 20 mins | Serves 4

Ingredients
- 1 tbsp. olive oil
- 2 onions , divided and meagerly cut
- 2 celery stems, finely chopped
- large bundle level leaf parsley , leaves and stalks isolated
- 2-3 tsp. paprika
- 200g broiled red pepper , depleted weight, thickly cut
- 400g can chopped tomato with garlic
- 400g white fish filet, cut into exceptionally large lumps
- barely any new mussels (discretionary)

Technique

1. Heat the oil in a container, at that point add the onions, celery and somewhat salt. Cover, at that point delicately fry until delicate, around 10 mins. Put the parsley stalks, a large portion of the leaves, oil and preparing into a food processor and whizz to a paste. Add this and the paprika to the relaxed onions, broiling for a couple of mins. Tip in the peppers and tomatoes with a sprinkle of water; at that point stew for 10 mins until the sauce has decreased.
2. Lay the fish and mussels on top of the sauce, put a cover on, and at that point stew for 5 mins until the fish is simply chipping and the mussels have opened – dispose of any that stay shut. Tenderly mix the fish into the sauce, season, at that point serve in bowls.
3. Formula TIPS
4. On the off chance that YOU WANT TO USE A SLOW COOKER...
5. Leave this stew to implant for more. Whizz the parsley stalks, a large portion of the leaves, oil and preparing in a food processor. Add this to the onions, celery, paprika, peppers and tomatoes in the slow cooker pot. Cook on Low for 8-10 hours. Settle the mussels in the sauce and dissipate the fish on top. Re-cover and cook on High for 30 mins 60 minutes. Dispose of any unopened mussels, mix the fish into the sauce at that point serve.
6. Works out positively For
7. Peach and almond crunch

5. Creamy veggie korma

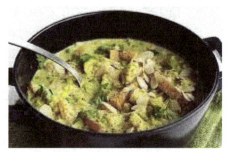

Prep: 15 mins | Cook: 30 mins | Serves 4

Ingredients
- 1 tbsp. vegetable oil
- 1 onion, finely chopped
- 3 cardamom cases, slammed
- 2 tsp. each ground cumin and coriander
- ½ tsp. ground turmeric
- 1 green bean stew, deseeded (whenever wanted) and finely chopped
- 1 garlic clove, squashed
- thumb-size piece ginger, finely chopped
- 800g blended vegetable, like carrots, cauliflower, potato and corvette, chopped
- 300-500ml hot vegetable stock
- 200g frozen peas
- 200ml yogurt
- 2 tbsp. ground almonds (discretionary)
- Make it non-veggie
- ½ little crude chicken bosom per divide
- To serve
- toasted chipped almonds, chopped coriander, basmati rice or naan bread

Strategy
1. Heat the oil in a large dish. Cook onion with the dry flavors over a low heat for 5-6 mins until the onion is light brilliant. Add the bean stew, garlic and ginger and cook for 1 min, at that point toss in the blended vegetables and cook for a further 5 mins.
2. Gap the blend fittingly between two dishes if serving veggie lovers and meat eaters. Slash the chicken into little pieces and mix into one dish. Add the stock, splitting between the dish properly, and stew for 10 mins (if just cooking the veggie rendition in one skillet, utilize 300ml stock; if splitting between two container, add 250ml to each). Gap the peas, if fundamental, and add, cooking for 3 mins more until the veg are delicate and the chicken is cooked through.
3. Eliminate from the heat and mix through the yogurt and ground almonds, if using. Serve sprinkled with the toasted almonds and coriander, with basmati rice or naan bread as an afterthought.
4. Formula TIPS
5. On the off chance that YOU WANT TO USE A SLOW COOKER...
6. On the off chance that you need to make the vegan rendition of this curry in a slow cooker, right off the bat cook off the onions with the dry flavors in a griddle for 5-6 mins. Add the bean stew, garlic and ginger and cook for 1 moment, at that point tip into your slow cooker. Toss in the vegetables and 400ml stock, cover and cook on Low for 4 hours until

the potatoes are delicate. Mix in the peas, yogurt and ground almonds with preparing, represent 5 minutes at that point fill in as above.
7. Works out in a good way For
8. One skillet fiery rice

6. Slow cooker lamb kolifto

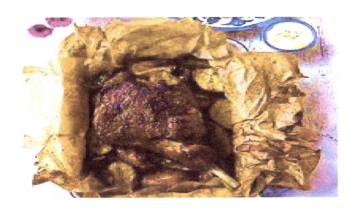

5 Hours + Marinating Serves 4

Ingredients
- Lemon 1 enormous, squeezed
- Extra-virgin olive oil 100ml
- Dry white wine 175ml
- Dark peppercorns squashed to make ½ tsp.
- Garlic 4 cloves, stripped and left entirety
- Dried oregano 2 tsp.
- Ground cumin 1 tsp.
- Sheep shanks 4
- Ocean salt drops 1 tsp.
- Ready tomato 1 enormous, cut into quarters
- Cinnamon stick 1
- Waxy potatoes 750g, stripped and cut into reduced down 3D squares
- Level leaf parsley a modest bunch, generally chopped

Directions:
1. Put the lemon juice, 2 tbsp. oil, wine, pepper, garlic, oregano and cumin into a blender and whizz. Put the shanks into a bowl, pour over the marinade and back rub well to cover. Cover and chill for at any rate 1 hour yet ideally overnight.
2. Heat the slow cooker to high or low, contingent upon wanted cooking time.
3. Put the meat, marinade, salt, tomato and cinnamon stick into the slow cooker. Cover with the top and cook for 3-4 hours on high, or 6-8 hours on low until totally delicate.
4. At the point when the sheep is cooked through and totally delicate, earthy colored the potatoes in 3 tbsp. of olive oil in a griddle over a medium-high heat until they start to shading and relax.
5. Eliminate the sheep from the slow cooker, put on a plate and cover firmly with foil.
6. Add the seared potatoes to the slow cooker and blend well. Cover and keep cooking for an additional 45 minutes-1 hour or until the potatoes are cooked and delicate. Add the sheep back to the slow cooker to heat through again. Check the flavoring, adding more if vital.
7. Present with hard bread and a green serving of mixed greens.

7. Slow-cooked duck legs in Port with celeriac gratin

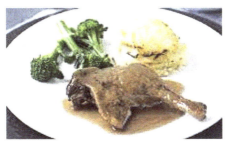

Cook: 2 hrs. and 30 mins | Prep 15 mins + infusing | Serves 2

Ingredients
- 2 duck legs
- 2 carrots , generally chopped
- 1 little onion , generally chopped
- 1 tbsp. plain flour
- 1 cove leaf
- 1 star anise
- 2 cloves
- 2 strips orange skin (with a potato peeler)
- 150ml port
- 500ml chicken stock
- For the gratin
- 100ml milk
- 100ml twofold cream
- 1 garlic clove , crushed
- 1 rosemary branch
- 25g margarine , in addition to extra for lubing
- ¼ little celeriac (about 100g), quartered and meagerly cut
- 1 little potato , meagerly cut

- ground parmesan , for sprinkling
- occasional vegetables , to serve

Technique
1. Heat oven to 160C/140C fan/gas 3. Put the duck legs in a flameproof goulash set over a medium heat. Brown all finished, at that point eliminate from the goulash and put away. Pour off everything except 1 tbsp. of the fat, leave more fat in the skillet on the off chance that you are multiplying or significantly increasing (save the depleted fat for your Christmas roasties). Add the carrots and onion to the goulash and cook for 5-10 mins or until beginning to caramelize. Mix in the flour and cook for 1 min more. Return the duck alongside the excess ingredients. Bring to a stew, at that point cover with a top and put in the oven for 2 hrs.
2. In the interim, set up the gratin. Put the milk, cream, garlic and rosemary in a dish set over a low heat. Bring to a delicate stew for 5 mins, at that point eliminate from the heat and leave to implant for 30 mins. Oil 2 ramekins (about 8cm breadth, 5cm profound). Mastermind the celeriac and potato cuts in the ramekins, preparing the layers as you go. Eliminate the garlic and rosemary from the milk, pour over the veg, at that point dab with spread. Cover firmly with thwart and prepare with the duck for 1½ hrs.
3. When cooked, eliminate the duck and gratins from the oven. To freeze the duck, cool, at that point pack into a cooler holder, pushing the

duck under the sauce. On the off chance that it doesn't cover it, lay stick film on top. Use inside 2 months. Defrost in the ice chest, at that point reheat in the meal and complete from Step 4. Increment oven to 220C/200C fan/gas 7. Put a hefty can on top of each foil-wrapped gratin and represent 15-20 mins, or chill like this until required. When squeezed, turn the gratins out onto a heating plate, sprinkle with a little Parmesan and prepare for 20 mins until brilliant.

4. In the interim, eliminate the duck legs from the goulash, strain the cooking fluid into a perfect container and bring to a fast bubble. Diminish the sauce significantly until thickened and polished. Add the duck legs and heat through. Put a duck leg on each plate with a little sauce spooned over the top. Present with the gratins and occasional veg.

8. Slow-cooked Greek Easter lamb with lemons, olives & bay

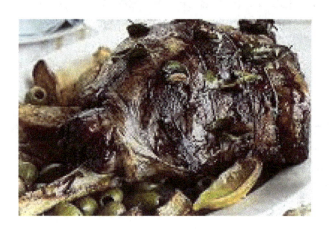

Prep: 20 mins | Cook: 4 hrs. and 30 mins | plus resting | Serves 6

Ingredients
- 1 garlic bulb , isolated into cloves, half stripped and cut, half unpeeled
- 8-10 new inlet leaves
- 3 lemons , cut into quarters lengthways
- 2 ½kg leg of sheep
- 50ml Greek additional virgin olive oil , in addition to 4 tbsp. for the potatoes
- 1 tsp. ground cinnamon
- 1kg Cypriot potatoes , stripped and quartered lengthways (in the event that you can't track down these, any large, waxy assortment is fine – attempt Desiree)
- 140g Greek Kalkidis olives (or other large hollowed green olives)
- 125ml red or dry white wine

Technique

1. Heat oven to 220C/200C fan/gas 7. Mastermind the unpeeled garlic cloves, 3 straight leaves and the lemon quarters in a large broiling dish and cover with 200ml virus water. Sit the sheep on top, shower with the olive oil and focus on everything over.
2. Using a little sharp blade, cut little cuts in the sheep skin, at that point fold the excess stripped and cut garlic and inlet leaves into these cuts.
3. Season the sheep well and sprinkle over the cinnamon. Cover firmly with foil and spot in the oven. Promptly diminish the oven temperature to 150C/130C fan/gas 2. Leave to cook for 4 hrs., skimming the fat from the juices and eliminating the foil for the last 30 mins of cooking.
4. After 1 hr., put the potato wedges in a large broiling tin, coat those in 4 tbsp. olive oil and season well. Broil in the oven with the sheep for 11/2-2 hrs.
5. Move the cooked sheep to a large part of foil wrap firmly and leave to rest for 20-30 mins. Check the potatoes are cooked (on the off chance that you need to, turn the oven up to 220C/200C fan/gas 7 to get done with cooking). Add the olives and wine to the container juices, stew them and keep warm until prepared to cut. Serve the sheep thickly cut with the olives, potatoes and Tahini and lemon sauce (see 'works out in a good way for'), with the meat juices pored over without a second to spare.

6. Formula TIPS
7. ADD A GARLIC HIT
8. For an additional hit of garlic, tenderly press the broiled (unpeeled) garlic cloves from the lower part of the dish with the rear of a spoon while the sheep rests. Blend the garlic into the dish juices prior to pouring over the meat.
9. Works out positively For
10. Tahini and lemon sauce
11. Spinach rice
12. Goliath spread bean stew

9. Slow-cooked celeriac with pork & orange

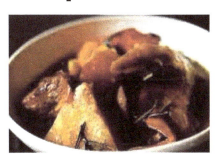

Total time3 hrs. | Ready in 2½-3 hrs. including 2 hours in the oven | More effort | Serves 2

Ingredients
- 3 leeks , managed and washed
- 2 carrots , stripped
- 3 tbsp. olive oil
- 900g boneless pork , cut into large stewing pieces (shoulder is an ideal sliced to utilize)
- 2 little or 1 large celeriac (about 1kg/2lb 4oz), stripped and diced into large pieces
- 2 garlic cloves , chopped
- 200ml dry white wine
- 200ml chicken stock
- squeeze and zing of 1 orange (eliminate the orange zing with a potato peeler)
- 2 tsp. soy sauce
- large twig of rosemary
- dried up bread , to serve

Strategy

1. Preheat the oven to fan 120C/regular 140C/gas 1. Cut every leek into around five pieces, hack the carrots into pieces similar size as the leeks. Heat a large, lidded, flameproof meal dish on the hob until it's hot. Add 2 tbsp. of the olive oil at that point cautiously tip the pork into the meal and leave it several minutes to brown. Mix once, at that point leaves for several minutes. Using an opened spoon, move the meat to a plate. Pour the remainder of the oil into the dish, tip in the leeks, carrots and celeriac and fry for 3-4 minutes, mixing, until they begin to brown. Add the garlic and fry briefly more.
2. Mix the pork and any juices into the vegetables, at that point pour in the wine, stock, squeezed orange and soy sauce. Toss in the rosemary and orange zing, season with salt and pepper, give it a mix, and at that point carry everything to the bubble.
3. Cover the dish, move it to the oven and cook for 2 hours, mixing following 60 minutes. Cook until the pork is delicate and the leeks self-destruct when pushed with a spoon. (It would now be able to be left to cool and afterward frozen for as long as multi month.) Leave to represent at any rate 10 minutes, at that point spoon into bowls. Present with hard bread to absorb each one of those juices.

10. Slow cooker chickpea Dahl

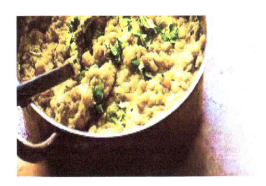

2 Hours 30 Minutes + Proving Serves 8

Ingredients
- sunflower oil
- onions 2 large, slashed
- ginger 50g, peeled and grated
- Ground cumin 1 tbsp.
- Ground coriander 1 tbsp.
- nigella seeds 1 tbsp., plus more for the naans
- Medium curry powder 1 tbsp.
- Turmeric 1 tsp.
- red split lentils 300g
- chana Dahl (dried split chickpeas) 500g
- coconut milk 2 x 400g tins
- NAANS
- fast-action dried yeast 7g
- natural yogurt 100g
- strong white bread flour 500g, plus more for dusting
- Fine salt 1½ tsp.

- clarified butter or ghee

DIRECTIONS:
1. To make the naans, blend the yeast and yogurt in with 250ml warm water. Put the flour and salt in a bowl and bit by bit mix in the yeast blend until it meets up as a batter. Tip out onto the work surface and massage for 10 minutes, or 5 minutes in a blender with the mixture snare, until smooth. Put into a perfect bowl, cover with oiled Clingfilm and leave for 2 hours, or until multiplied in size.
2. Heat 1 tbsp. oil in a huge skillet, and fry the onion and ginger until truly delicate. Mix in the flavors, cook for brief at that point add the lentils and chana Dahl. Add the coconut milk, 800ml water and some flavoring. Bring to a stew, go down to a low heat and cook for 1½ hours, covered, blending delicately from time to time, adding more water if necessary. To freeze, cool the Dahl totally, tip into compartments and put in the cooler.
3. At the point when the mixture is prepared, manipulate it momentarily on a softly floured work surface. Cut into 8 pieces and carry everyone out to an oval until they done spring back. Lay onto oiled preparing sheets, cover with oiled Clingfilm and leave for 30 minutes until puffy.
4. Heat the oven to 240C/fan 220C/gas 9. Heat another preparing sheet in the oven. Move the naans, two all at once, onto the hot preparing sheet. Cook for 5-10 minutes until the batter begins to bubble and the base looks brilliant.

Press them tenderly back down on the off chance that they've domed to an extreme. Cool under a perfect tea towel, at that point exclusively envelop by foil and freeze.

5. To reheat, thaw out the Dahl in the cooler short-term, and leave the naans on the work surface to come to room temperature. Heat the oven to 220C/fan 200C/gas 7. Put the Dahl into a dish with a sprinkle of water, bring to a stew and cook until steaming hot. Put the naans on a heating sheet, sprinkle with a little water and reheat in the oven for 5 minutes or until warmed through. Brush the naans with explained margarine or ghee, and disperse over some nigella seeds to serve.

6. Put all the Dahl ingredients and 800ml water in a slow cooker. Cook on high for 3 1/2 – 4 hours until the lentils are delicate.

11. Caramelised squash & spinach lasagna

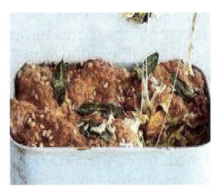

Prep: 25 mins | Cook: 1 hr. and 40 mins | plus cooling | Serves 6

Ingredients
- 1 medium butternut squash, stripped, seeds eliminated and cut into 2cm 3D squares (1.2kg arranged weight)
- 3 garlic cloves, unpeeled
- modest bunch of sage leaves
- 1 tbsp. olive oil, in addition to a little extra
- 600g new spinach
- 12-15 lasagne sheets
- 125g ball mozzarella, torn or cut into little pieces
- 40g pine nuts
- For the white sauce
- 70g margarine
- 70g flour
- 800ml milk
- 250g mascarpone

- 50g parmesan (or veggie lover elective), ground
- grinding of nutmeg

Strategy
1. Heat the oven to 200C/180C fan/gas 6. Tip the squash and garlic into a large cooking tin or dish (you can utilize a similar one to amass the lasagne to save money on cleaning up – our own was 35 x 40cm and 5cm profound). Tear more than 4-5 sage leaves, shower with the oil and season well, and at that point throw to cover. Cook for 40-50 mins, moving the squash around more than once, until delicate and caramelized. Crush the garlic from the skins and pound with the squash, leaving a couple of stout pieces for surface.
2. In the mean time, make the white sauce. Soften the spread in a large pot, and mix in the flour to make a sandy paste. Sprinkle a little milk into the dish, blending constantly to forestall bumps. Continue to add more milk, a little at a time, until the paste diminishes to a smooth, rich sauce and the milk has all been utilized. Stew for 1 min more. Mix in the mascarpone and a large portion of the parmesan. Season well and mesh in a liberal measure of nutmeg.
3. Tip the spinach into a colander and pour over a kettleful of bubbling water to shrink (do this in clumps). When sufficiently cool to deal with, crush the spinach over the colander to eliminate the water, at that point season and generally cleave.

4. Eliminate half of the squashed garlicky squash from the cooking tin and put away on a plate. Spread the excess squash out over the base of the tin or dish you mean to serve the lasagne in. Spoon over about a fourth of the sauce, at that point top with a solitary layer of lasagne sheets, snapping them to fill any holes. Make an even layer of spinach on top of the pasta, and top with another quarter of the sauce, more pasta, squash, sauce, pasta lastly the excess white sauce.
5. Disperse over the leftover parmesan, the mozzarella and pine nuts. On the off chance that the oven is off, heat to 200C/180C fan/gas 6 and cook the lasagne for 30 mins. Rub some additional oil more than 5 or 6 sage leaves, place them on top of the lasagne and get back to the oven for another 15-20 mins until brilliant and percolating. Leave to cool for 5 mins prior to serving.
6. Works out in a good way For
7. Slow-cooked stout meat lasagne
8. Green plate of mixed greens with olive dressing
9. Green plate of mixed greens with buttermilk dressing.

12. Lamb bhuna

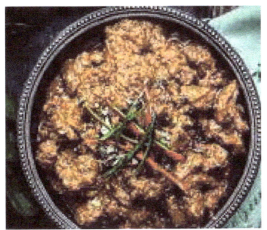

Prep: 30 mins | Cook: 1 hr. and 40 min| plus at least 1 hr. marinating | More effort | Serves 4

Ingredients
- 600g sheep neck filet or shoulder, cut into large lumps
- For the marinade
- 6 garlic cloves, finely ground
- thumb-sized piece of ginger, stripped and finely ground
- 2 tbsp. malt vinegar
- ½ tsp. ground cinnamon
- 1 tbsp. sunflower oil
- For the sauce
- 3 tbsp. sunflower oil, in addition to some extra if necessary
- 2 onions, finely chopped
- 10 curry leaves
- 2 dried chilies, or ½ tsp. stew drops
- 1 tsp. cumin seeds
- 1 tsp. mustard seeds

- 1 tsp. ground coriander
- ½ tsp. fenugreek seeds or ground fenugreek
- 1 tbsp. tomato purée
- 400g can chopped tomatoes
- 1 tsp. gram masala

Strategy
1. To make the marinade, consolidate the ingredients with a large touch of salt in a large bowl. Throw in the sheep, cover and marinate for 1 hr. at room temperature, or chill for the time being.
2. For the sauce, heat the oil in a flameproof meal and fry the onions for 10 mins, blending until delicate and brilliant. Shower in more oil if the dish gets dry. Add the curry leaves and chilies and fry for a couple of moments, at that point add the flavors and cook for 5 mins more until the onions begin to caramelize.
3. Tip in the sheep alongside the marinade and turn the heat to high. Cook, mixing, for 5 mins until the sheep browns. Add the tomato purée and cook for 1 min, at that point mix in the tomatoes and 100ml water. Bring to a stew, decrease the heat, cover and cook, mixing every so often, for 1 hr. 20 mins until the sheep is delicate.
4. Reveal and cook for 8-10 mins more until the sauce has decreased and thickened. Eliminate from the heat, mix in the garam masalaa and season. Will keep chilled for as long as three days or frozen for a very long time.
5. Works out in a good way For
6. Carrot pakoras

7. Paneer and chickpea fry
8. Fast and puffy flatbreads

13. Herb-scented slow-roasted rib of beef

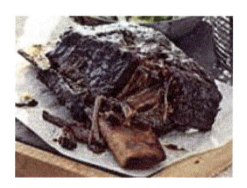

Prep: 30 mins | Cook: 5 hrs. | Plus at least 3 hrs. to bring to room temperature and resting | More effort | Serves 10

Ingredients
- 3-bone rib of hamburger joint (around 3-3.5kg)
- 4 garlic cloves , left entire however slammed once
- 4 rosemary twigs
- ½ pack thyme
- small bunch inlet leaves
- 4 allspice berries
- 4 cloves
- 1 tsp. dark peppercorns
- 200ml red wine
- 1 tbsp. plain flour
- For the coating
- 2 tbsp. Bovril
- 2 tbsp. Dijon mustard
- 1 tbsp. dark remedy

Technique
1. Remove the hamburger from the cooler and surrender it to come to temperature short-term or for at any rate three hours. Tip the garlic and every one of the spices and flavors into a large simmering tin and, using a blow light or under a hot flame broil, burn the spices until they begin to seethe (in the event that using a barbecue to do this, don't leave it unattended), leave to cool marginally.
2. Heat oven to 100C/80C fan/gas ¼. Rub a tbsp. of salt over the meat; at that point sit the joint on top of the spices. Pour over the wine; at that point firmly tent the tin two or three sheets of extra-wide foil. Cook in the oven for 1 hr., at that point lessen the temperature to 70C/50C fan (on the off chance that you have a gas oven, don't change the temperature), and slow dish for 3 hrs. more.
3. Eliminate the foil, at that point embed a computerized test into the center of the joint – when the temperature stretches around 60C, it's prepared. In the event that the meat isn't up to temperature, increment oven to 150C/130C fan/gas 2, and meal with the foil off, checking the temperature each 15 mins. While the hamburger is cooking, make the coating by whisking every one of the ingredients together.
4. At the point when the hamburger is cooked, eliminate from the oven and increment the temperature to 230C/210C fan/gas 8. Return the hamburger to the oven for 5 mins to fresh and rankle the fat, at that point liberally brush

the coating everywhere on the joint and get back to the oven for 5 mins until tacky and slightly singed – watch out for it, as it will consume effectively at this stage. Lift the meat onto a slashing load up and leave to rest for 20 mins.
5. To make a herby sauce, put the broiling tin over a low heat and mix in the flour to make a gloopy paste. Include any excess coating, at that point cautiously pour in 500ml bubbling water. Bubble for a couple of moments, at that point strain into a little dish and keep warm. Serve the hamburger in thick cuts, with sauce as an afterthought.
6. Formula TIPS
7. COOK MEAT PERFECTLY
8. For more extraordinary meat, focus on an inner temperature of 55C while slow cooking. For all around done, focus on 75C.

14. Slow-roasted courgettes with fennel & orzo

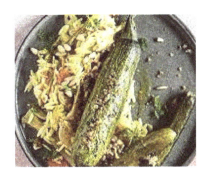

Prep: 25 mins | Cook: 2 hrs. and 10 mins | Easy | Serves 2

Ingredients
- touch of saffron
- 1/2 bulb of fennel , cut
- 100g cherry tomatoes , split
- 1 straight leaf
- 2 tbsp. olive oil
- spot of dried stew drops
- 120ml dry white wine
- 4-6 child to medium-sized courgettes
- 1 lemon , zested
- 50g sourdough breadcrumbs
- 200g orzo
- 1 tbsp. pine nuts , toasted
- 1 tbsp. ricotta
- modest bunch of dill

Technique

1. Put the saffron in a little bowl and cover with 1/2 tbsp. of bubbling water. Heat oven to 180C/160C fan/gas 4. Put the fennel in a broiling tin with the tomatoes and sound leaf, shower over some oil, season and throw along with the bean stew drops. Pour over the wine. Prick the courgettes done with a fork and spot on top of the fennel. Sprinkle with somewhat more oil, at that point season and cover with foil.
2. Cook for 1/2 - 2 hrs., turning the courgettes partially through, eliminating the foil for the last 5 mins. The courgettes ought to be delicate. Lift the courgettes from the container and put away.
3. In the mean time, heat 1 tbsp. olive oil in a skillet over a medium heat. Add a large portion of the lemon zing and breadcrumbs, and tenderly fry until the bread is brilliant and crunchy. Put away.
4. Cook the orzo in a skillet of bubbling water until still somewhat firm, at that point channel. Throw with the fennel, tomatoes, pine nuts, the saffron and its water. Season.
5. Split the orzo among plates and add a large portion of the ricotta to each, shower with olive oil and sprinkle with ocean salt. Top with the courgettes and disperse over the breadcrumbs, remaining lemon zing and branches of dill.
6. Works out in a good way For
7. Tomato, burrata and expansive bean salad
8. Squashed cannellini beans with shriveled greens and seared artichokes

9. Singed nectarine and prosciutto panzanella.

15. Bourbon & honey-glazed brisket with soured cream & chive mash

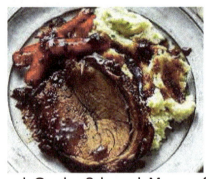

Prep: 15 mins | Cook: 8 hrs. | More effort | Serves 6-8

Ingredients
- 3 tbsp. vegetable oil
- 2-2½ kg piece meat brisket , rolled and tied (request that your butcher do this for you)
- 1 tbsp. smoked paprika
- 1 tbsp. English mustard powder
- 2 tsp. dried onion powder
- 1 tsp. ground cinnamon
- squeeze dried ground cloves
- 6 tbsp. light brown delicate sugar
- 100g nectar
- 50ml whiskey bourbon, in addition to 2 tbsp.
- 2 red onions , cut
- 4 sound leaves

- 4-6 little carrots , stripped and split or quartered lengthways or 300g Chantenay carrots
- 100ml red wine vinegar
- For the soured cream and chive pound
- 4-6 large preparing potatoes , unpeeled
- 250g soured cream
- 75g spread , in addition to extra to serve
- sprinkle of milk
- little pack chives , chopped

Strategy

1. Heat 1 tbsp. oil in a large, profound flameproof broiling tin or in your largest flameproof meal dish. Season the meat well and burn in the tin until pleasantly browned all finished, adding the leftover oil to the dish if necessary. Then, blend the paprika, mustard powder, onion powder, cinnamon, cloves, 2 tbsp. sugar, 2 tbsp. nectar and 2 tbsp. of the bourbon in a little bowl with a liberal measure of salt and pepper. Lift out the hamburger and disperse the onions and inlet leaves over the base of the dish, pour in 100ml water and set the meat back on top. Brush the flavor paste everywhere on the meat. Will keep chilled for as long as a day.
2. Heat oven to 150C/130C fan/gas 2. Wrap the tin firmly in a couple of sheets of foil, or cover with a top, and heat for 6-7 hrs., turning more than once during cooking, spooning the juices over the meat and garnish up with a sprinkle more water if the lower part of the dish is dry.

3. Increment the temperature to 200C/180C fan/gas 6. Throw the carrots with the onions around the meat, season at that point cover again with the foil. Penetrate the potatoes a couple of times each and place on the rack underneath the hamburger. Cook for a further 45 mins.
4. Then, pour the leftover sugar, bourbon, nectar and vinegar into a container. In the event that there is bunches of fluid in the tin, add the majority of this as well (yet leave some so the meat doesn't dry out). Season and air pocket to make a tacky coating. Uncover the meat and carrots, brush with the bourbon coating and cook for another 15 mins until the meat is dull, lustrous and delicate, and the carrots and potatoes are delicate. Eliminate from the oven, cover the meat freely with foil and leave to rest for 15 mins.
5. Put the potatoes in a bowl and, when sufficiently cool to deal with, use kitchen scissors to cut them into pieces – you need to save the skin in the pound for additional flavor however any large pieces will be chewy so attempt to separate it however much as could reasonably be expected with the scissors, at that point squash well with a potato masher. Add the soured cream, margarine, milk and the vast majority of the chives, season truly well and crush once more. Move to a bowl and top with a handle of spread and the excess chives. To serve, either cut into thick, delicate cuts or shred the meat with two forks, disposing of any string as you go. Present with

the crush, carrots and onions and spoon over the juices.
6. Works out positively For
7. Thai green curry cook chicken
8. Stuffed butternut squash
9. Darkened dish salmon with avocado and mango salsa.

16. Sweet corn fritters with slow-cooked tomatoes

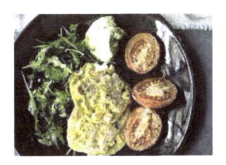

Prep: 30 mins | Cook: 40 mins | Easy | Serves 4

Ingredients
- 6 large, ready plum tomatoes , divided
- spot of sugar
- avocado cream, (see lower part of pag) to serve
- For the wastes

- 450g sweet corn - utilize new, frozen (thawed out) or canned (depleted)
- 175g plain flour
- 1 tsp. heating powder
- 2 eggs and 2 yolks, beaten
- 125ml milk
- 25g margarine, softened
- 2 spring onions, finely chopped
- ½ red bean stew, deseeded and finely diced
- juice ½ lime
- 25g feta cheddar, disintegrated
- 1 tbsp. each chopped basil and parsley
- olive oil, for fricasseeing
- For the olive serving of mixed greens
- 200g large dark olives, stoned and chopped
- 4 large modest bunches rocket
- sprinkle olive oil
- crush lime juice

Technique

1. Heat oven to 150C/130C fan/gas 2. Season the tomatoes; add a spot of sugar and meal for around 40 mins. This will focus all their regular pleasantness and flavor.
2. In the case of using new corn, strip away the husks, cut the parts off with a blade, and at that point cook in bubbling water for 4-5 mins. Channel. Filter the flour and preparing powder into a bowl, making a well in the middle. Add the eggs, yolks and a large portion of the milk. Beat until smooth; at that point slowly rush in the excess milk and margarine. Crease in the corn, spring onions, bean stew, lime juice, feta

and spices. Season, remembering the feta is somewhat pungent.
3. Heat and delicately oil a weighty based skillet. Drop 2-3 loaded tbsp. of the combination into the container and fry over a medium heat for around 3 mins each side, or until brilliant brown and cooked through. Move to the oven and rehash with the leftover player – makes around 16. They will save well like this for a couple of hours, in the event that you need to make them ahead.
4. For the plate of mixed greens, blend the olives, spices and rocket together. Shower with oil and lime juice. Serve the wastes with the plate of mixed greens, tomato parts and avocado cream.
5. Formula TIPS
6. AVOCADO CREAM
7. Put 2 medium stripped and generally chopped avocados, juice 1 large lime, ½ little garlic clove squashed and ½ tbsp. olive oil in a food processor. Whizz to a smooth purée and overlap in 2 tbsp. crème fraîche. Taste and season, adding more lime juice in the event that you figure the flavor could be somewhat more honed.

17. Venetian duck ragu

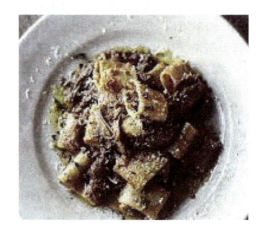

Prep: 15 mins| Cook: 2 hrs. and 30 mins | Easy | Serves 6

Ingredients
- 1 tbsp. olive oil
- 4 duck legs
- 2 onions, finely chopped
- 2 fat garlic cloves, squashed
- 2 tsp. ground cinnamon
- 2 tsp. plain flour
- 250ml red wine
- 2 x 400g jars chopped tomatoes
- 1 chicken stock solid shape, made up to 250ml
- 3 rosemary branches, leaves picked and chopped
- 2 straight leaves
- 1 tsp. sugar
- 2 tbsp. milk
- 600g paccheri or pappardelle pasta
- parmesan, ground, to serve

Strategy

1. Heat the oil in a large container. Add the duck legs and brown on all sides for around 10 mins. Eliminate to a plate and put away. Add the onions to the container and cook for 5 mins until relaxed. Add the garlic and cook for a further 1 min, at that point mix in the cinnamon and flour and cook for a further min. Return the duck to the dish, add the wine, tomatoes, stock, spices, sugar and preparing. Bring to a stew, at that point bring down the heat, cover with a top and cook for 2 hrs., blending from time to time.
2. Cautiously lift the duck legs out of the sauce and spot on a plate – they will be delicate so do whatever it takes not to lose any of the meat. Pull off and dispose of the fat, at that point shred the meat with 2 forks and dispose of the bones. Add the meat back to the sauce with the milk and stew, revealed, for a further 10-15 mins while you cook the pasta.
3. Cook the pasta adhering to pack guidelines, at that point channel, holding some the pasta water, and add the pasta to the ragu. Mix to cover all the pasta in the sauce and cook for 1 min more, adding a sprinkle of cooking fluid on the off chance that it looks dry. Present with ground Parmesan, in the event that you like.
4. Works out positively For
5. Panna cotta with apricot compote
6. Tart fennel and rocket salad

18. Low 'n' slow rib steak with Cuban mojo salsa

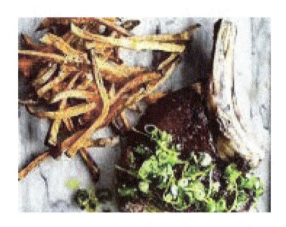

Preparation and cooking time | Prep: 20 mins | Cook: 3 hrs. and 20 mins | More effort | Serves 2
Ingredients
- 1 rib steak on the bone or côte du boeuf (about 800g)
- 1 tbsp. rapeseed oil
- 1 garlic clove
- 2 thyme branches
- 25g margarine , chopped into little pieces
- yam fries
- a dressed plate of mixed greens , to serve
- For the magic salsa
- 2 limes
- 1 little orange
- ½ little bundle mint , finely chopped
- little bundle coriander , finely chopped
- 4 spring onions , finely chopped
- 1 little garlic clove , squashed

- 1 fat green bean stew , finely chopped
- 4 tbsp. additional virgin rapeseed oil or olive oil

Technique
1. Leave the hamburger at room temperature for around 1 hr. before you cook it. Heat oven to 60C/40C fan/gas 1/4 on the off chance that you like your meat medium uncommon, or 65C/45C fan/gas 1/4 for medium. (Cooking at these low temperatures will be more precise in an electric oven than in a gas one. In the case of using gas, put the oven on the most reduced setting you have, and know that the cooking time might be more limited.)
2. Put the unseasoned hamburger in a weighty based ovenproof skillet. Cook in the oven for 3 hrs. undisturbed.
3. Then, make the salsa. Zing the limes and orange into a bowl. Slice each down the middle and spot, cut-side down, in a hot skillet. Cook for a couple of mins until the organic products are burned, at that point crushes the juice into the bowl. Add different ingredients and season well.
4. At the point when the hamburger is cooked, it should look dry on a superficial level, and dull pink in shading. On the off chance that you have a meat thermometer, test the inside temperature – it ought to be 58-60C. Eliminate the dish from the oven and set over a high heat on the hob. Add the oil and singe the meat on the two sides for a couple of mins until caramelized. Singe the fat for a couple of mins as well. Crush the garlic clove with the

impact point of your hand and add this to the container with the thyme and spread. At the point when the spread is frothing, spoon it over the meat and cook for another 1-2 mins. Move the meat to a warm plate, cover with foil, and leave to rest for 5-10 mins. Cut away from the bone and into cuts prior to presenting with the salsa, fries and salad.

5. Works out positively For
6. Chimichurri sauce
7. Heated thin fries
8. Yam fries

19. Slow-roast pork rolls with apple chili chutney

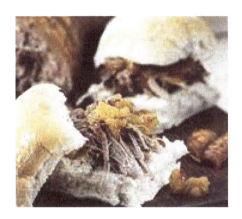

Prep: 15 mins | Cook: 6 hrs. | Easy| Serves 6 - 8

Ingredients
- 2.5kg/5lb 8oz pork shoulder joint, scored and tied (we utilized a tied carvery joint from Waitrose, bone in one end and rolled and tied at opposite end)
- 2 tsp. thyme leaves
- 1 tsp. fennel seed
- 1 tbsp. olive oil
- buttered delicate bread moves , to serve
- For the apple stew chutney
- 1 tbsp. olive oil
- 2 onions , finely chopped
- 1-2 red chilies , deseeded and finely chopped
- 4 eating apples , stripped, cored and cut into little pieces
- 4 tbsp. juice vinegar
- 4 tbsp. caster sugar

- 1 thyme twig, leaves picked

Strategy
1. Heat oven to 240C/220C fan/gas 9. Sit the pork in a large cooking tin. In the event that the skin isn't as of now scored for you, score it with a little, sharp blade. Combine as one the thyme, fennel seeds, oil and 1 tsp. salt with a decent crushing of dark pepper. Rub this ludicrous and finishes of the pork. Broil for 30 mins, at that point cover the entire tin with a large sheet of foil, diminish the oven temperature to 140C/120C fan/gas 1 and return the pork to the oven for a further 5 hrs.
2. While the pork is cooking, make the chutney. Heat the oil in a large pot. Relax the onion and bean stew together for 10-15 mins. When delicate, mix in the apple lumps, vinegar and sugar with 50ml water. Cover and cook over a low heat for 15-20 mins, blending sporadically, until the apple is exceptionally delicate. Rush a large portion of the apple combination with a hand blender, or scoop half into a food processor and whizz until smooth, prior to mixing once more into the container with the leaves from the thyme twig.
3. Take the pork from the oven – the meat ought to be delicate – and increment the temperature to 240C/220C fan/gas 9. At the point when the oven has arrived at temperature, dispose of the foil and set the pork back in for 30 mins to fresh up the skin a bit. For truly fresh popping, eliminate the skin from the meat, envelop the meat by foil to keep warm, and return just the

skin to the oven for 30 mins. A few forks to shred the pork from the joint. Sandwich in delicate buttered moves with apple bean stew chutney, warm or at room temperature. Present with bits of fresh snapping as an afterthought.

20. Beef bourguignon with celeriac mash

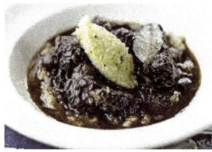

Prep: 20 mins |Cook:3 hrs. and 15 mins | Easy | Serves 4

Ingredients
- 1 tbsp. goose fat
- 600g shin meat, cut into large lumps
- 100g smoked dirty bacon, cut
- 350g shallot or pearl onions, stripped
- 250g chestnut mushrooms (around 20)
- 2 garlic cloves, cut
- 1 bouquet garni (see ability beneath)
- 1 tbsp. tomato purée
- 750ml jug red wine, Burgundy is acceptable
- For the celeriac pound
- 600g (around 1) celeriac
- 2 tbsp. olive oil, in addition to a glug
- 1 or 2 rosemary and thyme twigs
- 2 cove leaves
- 4 cardamom units

Strategy
1. Heat a large goulash dish and add 1 tbsp. goose fat.

2. Season 600g large lumps of shin hamburger and fry until brilliant brown, around 3-5 mins, at that point turn over and fry the opposite side until the meat is browned all finished, adding more fat if important. Do this in 2-3 clusters, moving the meat to a colander set over a bowl when browned.
3. In a similar skillet, fry 100g cut smoked smudgy bacon, 350g stripped shallots or pearl onions, 250g chestnut mushrooms, 2 cut garlic cloves and 1 bouquet garni until softly browned.
4. Blend in 1 tbsp. tomato purée and cook for a couple of mins, mixing the combination. This enhances the bourguignon and makes an incredible base for the stew. At that point return the meat and any depleted juices to the skillet and mix through.
5. Pour over 750ml container red wine and about 100ml water so the meat bounces up from the fluid, however isn't totally covered. Bring to the bubble and utilize a spoon to scratch the caramelized cooking juices from the lower part of the container – this will give the stew more flavors.
6. Heat oven to 150C/fan 130C/gas 2. Make a cartouche: detach a square of foil somewhat larger than the goulash, organize it in the skillet so it covers the highest point of the stew and trim away any abundance foil. Cook for 3 hrs.
7. On the off chance that the sauce looks watery, eliminate the meat and veg with an opened spoon, and put away. Cook the sauce over a

high heat for a couple of mins until the sauce has thickened a little, at that point returns the hamburger and vegetables to the dish.
8. To make the celeriac squash, strip 600g celeriac and cut into blocks. Heat 2 tbsp. olive oil in a large griddle. Tip in the celeriac and fry for 5 mins until it becomes brilliant. Season well with salt and pepper.
9. Mix in 1 or 2 branches of rosemary and thyme, 2 cove leaves and 4 cardamom cases, at that point pour over 200ml water, enough to almost cover the celeriac. Turn the heat to low, in part cover the container and leave to stew for 25-30 mins.
10. After 25-30 mins, the celeriac ought to be delicate and the majority of the water will have vanished. Channel away any excess water, at that point eliminate the spice branches, sound and cardamom units.
11. Daintily smash with a potato masher, at that point get done with a glug of olive oil and season to taste.
12. Spoon the hamburger bourguignon into serving bowls and spot a large spoonful of the celeriac pound on top. Enhancement with one of the narrows leaves, on the off chance that you like.
13. Formula TIPS
14. MAKE AHEAD
15. Attempt to make this dish a day ahead of time, at that point slowly reheat in the oven. You'll see that the flavors will truly grow for the time being and the dish will be more extravagant and more develop.

16. Skill - BOUQUET GARNI
17. To make a bouquet garni, utilize a piece of string to two or three rosemary, thyme and parsley twigs and a small bunch of inlet leaves. Eliminate from the dish toward the finish of cooking and dispose of.
18. Hamburger SHIN
19. Hamburger shin is an incredible cut for slow-cooking. It's acceptable worth and the waves of fat going through it guarantee that it doesn't dry out. You could likewise utilize wild hog, which gives a truly unique flavor.
20. TIP - PEELING ONIONS
21. To strip shallots or pearl onions rapidly, place in an astonish and pour bubbling water. Leave for a couple of moments, at that point channel and the skins will sneak off.
22. Works out positively For:
23. Irish soft drink bread

21. Slow cooked Ossobuco

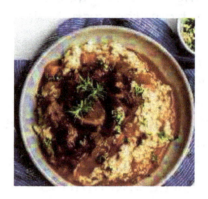

Prep tim2: 3 hours | Serves 2

Ingredients
- veal or meat shin 8 pieces around 4-5cm thick, cut across the bone (request that the butcher do this)
- plain flour 100g, all around prepared
- olive oil
- onions 2 enormous, finely chopped
- carrots 4, stripped and finely chopped
- celery 4 sticks, managed and finely chopped
- garlic 4 cloves, squashed
- white wine 300ml
- sound leaves 3
- thyme 3 twigs
- veal or chicken stock 1.5-2 liters
- GERMOLATA
- lemon 1, zested
- garlic 1 cloves, finely chopped
- level leaf parsley a little bundle, finely chopped

DIRECTION:
1. Heat the oven to 180C/fan 160C/gas 4. Season the veal pieces well, at that point delicately dust in the prepared flour.

2. Heat 2 tbsp. oil in a non-stick dish on a high heat, and fry the meat in groups for a couple of moments on each side until brilliant earthy colored. Move to a plate and rehash with the excess pieces. Add another tbsp. oil to the dish, on the off chance that you need to, while singing.
3. Lower the heat to medium and add tbsp. oil to the container in the event that you need to, add the onion, carrot, celery and a touch of salt. Fry for 10 minutes until exceptionally delicate and clear.
4. Add the garlic and fry for one more moment prior to pouring in the wine. Stew until decreased considerably, scraping up any pieces from the lower part of the skillet. Add the narrows leaves and thyme.
5. Move the meat, the veg and the fluid from the griddle to a huge goulash with a cover. Add the stock to simply cover the meat, season well and bring to a stew.
6. Cover with the top and move to the oven. Cook for 2 hours until the meat is truly delicate (you may require longer for hamburger shin).
7. Combine the gremolata ingredients as one with a touch of salt and dissipate over the ossobuco. Present with crush, polenta, or saffron risotto.

8. Instructions to store it: serve straight away, or leave to cool to room temperature and move to Tupperware boxes, and freeze. It will save for a half year. Defrost in the cooler expedite and reheat.

Conclusion

Thank you for going through recipes in this book. Slow cooker is easy to use and it just needs practice. Try the incredible recipes in this book and enjoy.
I wish you good luck!

CPSIA information can be obtained
at www.ICGtesting.com
Printed in the USA
BVHW092256250521
608096BV00004B/258